Asthma FOR DUMMIES®

POCKET EDITION

by William E. Berger, MD, MBA

Look for Pocket Editions on these other topics:

Allergies For Dummies, Pocket Edition
Anxiety & Depression For Dummies, Pocket Edition
Diabetes For Dummies, Pocket Edition
Dieting For Dummies, Pocket Edition
Heart Disease For Dummies, Pocket Edition
High Blood Pressure For Dummies, Pocket Edition
Menopause For Dummies, Pocket Edition
Migraines For Dummies, Pocket Edition

WILEY

Wiley Publishing, Inc.

Asthma For Dummies, Pocket Edition

Published by
Wiley Publishing, Inc.
111 River St.
Hoboken, NJ 07030-5774
www.wiley.com

For general information on our other products and services, please contact our Customer Care Department within the U.S. at 800-762-2974, outside the U.S. at 317-572-3993, or fax 317-572-4002.

For technical support, please visit www.wiley.com/techsupport.

Wiley also publishes its books in a variety of electronic formats. Some content that appears in print may not be available in electronic books.

Library of Congress Control Number: 2005936637

ISBN-13: 978-0-471-79233-8

ISBN-10: 0-471-79233-0

Manufactured in the United States of America

10 9 8 7 6 5 4 3 2 1

1O/SR/RS/QV/IN

Publisher's Acknowledgments

Project Editor: Georgette Beatty
Copy Editor: Sarah Faulkner
Composition Services: Indianapolis Composition Services Department
Cover Photo: © Spencer Rowell/Getty Images/Taxi

Table of Contents

Introduction

"I feel like I'm breathing through a straw." "Oh, my aching sinuses." "I can't stop coughing." If you've ever uttered words like these, you're not alone. Statements similar to these are some of the most frequent medical complaints that people in the United States and around the world report, and their complaints often describe asthma symptoms.

How are you feeling? Do you, or someone you know, think that having asthma means that feeling unwell is normal and that your condition can never improve? Unfortunately, many people answer yes to this question. However, the plain, simple, and accurate medical truth is this: Although no cure exists for asthma, when you receive effective, appropriate care from your doctor, combined with your motivated participation as a patient, you can lead a normal, active, and fulfilling life.

About This Book

I wrote this book to give you sound, up-to-date, practical advice, based on my 25-plus years of experience with numerous patients, about dealing with your asthma effectively and appropriately. For that reason, I structure this book so that you can jump to sections that most directly apply to your medical condition. You don't need to read this book from cover to cover, although I won't object if you do. (Be careful, though, because when you start reading, you may have a hard time putting it down!)

This book can also serve as a reference and source for information about the many facets of diagnosing, treating, and managing asthma. Although you may pick up this book for one aspect of asthma, you may realize later that other topics also apply to you or a loved one.

Don't worry about remembering where related subjects are in this book. I provide ample cross-references in every chapter that remind you where to look for the information you may need in other chapters or within other sections of the chapter that you're reading.

I intend the information in this book to empower you as a person with asthma, thus helping you to

✔ Set goals for your treatment

✔ Ensure that you receive the most appropriate and effective medical care for your condition

✔ Do your part as a patient by adhering to the treatment plan that you and your physician develop

Foolish Assumptions

I don't think I'm being too foolish, but I assume that you want substantive, scientifically accurate, relevant information about asthma, presented in everyday language, without a lot of medical mumbo-jumbo. In this book, you find straightforward explanations when I present important scientific aspects of asthma and use key medical terms.

If you've chosen to read my book, I know you're no dummy, so I'm willing to go out on a limb and make some further assumptions about you, dear reader:

- ✔ You or someone you care about suffers from asthma.
- ✔ You want to educate yourself about asthma as part of improving your medical condition (in consultation with your doctor, of course).
- ✔ You want to feel better.
- ✔ You really like doctors named Bill.

Icons Used in This Book

Throughout the book, you may notice the following icons. They're intended to alert you to the type of information I present in particular paragraphs. Here's what they mean:

 The Berger Bit icon represents me expressing my opinion.

 Myths and misconceptions abound about asthma. The Myth Buster icon indicates that I expose and correct mistaken beliefs that many people hold about asthma.

 The Remember icon indicates things you shouldn't forget, because you may find the information useful in the future. (Now, where did I put my car keys?)

 The See Your Doctor icon alerts you to matters that you should discuss with your physician.

 To give you as complete a picture as possible, I occasionally get into more complex details of medical science. The Technical Stuff icon lets you know that's what I'm doing so that you can delve into the topic further — or skip it. You don't have to read these paragraphs to understand the subject at hand. (However, reading the information marked with these icons may give you a better handle on managing your medical condition, as well as provide some great material for impressing friends at your next party.)

 You can find plenty of helpful information and advice in paragraphs marked with the Tip icon.

 A Warning icon advises you about potential problems, such as symptoms you shouldn't ignore or treatments that you may not want to undergo.

Where to Go from Here

Although you can read this book from cover to cover if you want, I suggest turning to the table of contents and finding the sections that apply to your immediate concern. Then begin reading your way to better management of your asthma.

If you want even more information on asthma, check out the full-size version of *Asthma For Dummies* — simply head to your local bookseller or go to www.dummies.com!

Chapter 1

Asthma 101

· ·

In This Chapter

▶ Identifying who has asthma and why

▶ Understanding the dimensions of asthma

▶ Connecting the dots from airways to asthma

▶ Diagnosing your condition

▶ Undertaking an asthma management plan

· ·

*A*sthma isn't a recurring chest cold, a psychological disorder, a minor annoyance, or a condition that you usually outgrow. It's a multifaceted, chronic, inflammatory airway disease of the lungs that causes breathing problems and that requires proper diagnosis, early and aggressive treatment, and effective long-term management.

Asthma is also unfortunately an ailment that many people — asthmatics themselves, family members, and even some doctors — may not recognize or may improperly diagnose, often as a chest cold or bronchitis.

Doctors don't yet clearly understand the origin of the airway inflammation that characterizes asthma. However, researchers have determined that this underlying inflammation often results in hyperresponsive ("twitchy"), constricted, and congested airways, which are increasingly liable to react to asthma triggers (see Chapter 3 for an extensive discussion of these triggers).

Understanding Who Gets Asthma and Why

The strongest predictor that an individual may develop asthma is a family history of allergies and asthma and/or *atopy,* an inherited tendency to develop hypersensitivities to allergic triggers. This tendency is almost always due to an overactive immune system that produces elevated levels of immunoglobulin E (IgE) antibodies to allergens. Two-thirds of asthma patients have a family member who also has the disease.

Most cases of asthma are of an allergic nature (known as *allergic asthma*), and usually begin to manifest during childhood, affecting boys more often than girls. In fact, asthma is the most common chronic disease of childhood. Other allergic disorders, such as food allergies, atopic dermatitis (allergic eczema), or allergic rhinitis (hay fever), which are also indicators of atopy in young children, can precede this form of the ailment, often referred to as childhood-onset asthma.

Adult-onset asthma, which is less common than childhood-onset asthma, develops in adults older than 40, more often in women. Atopy doesn't appear to play a role in these cases. Rather, adult-onset asthma more often seems to be triggered by various nonallergic mechanisms, including sinusitis, upper respiratory infections, nasal polyps, gastroesophageal reflux disease (GERD), sensitivities to aspirin and related nonsteroidal anti-inflammatory drugs (NSAIDs), as well as occupational exposures to chemicals, such as those found in fumes, gases, resins, dust, and insecticides. However, many episodes seem to occur spontaneously without known triggers.

Keep these points in mind about asthma:

- ✔ Important symptoms of asthma in infancy and early childhood include persistent coughing, wheezing, and recurring or lingering chest colds.

- ✔ Inflammation of the airways is the single most important underlying factor in asthma. If you have asthma, your symptoms may come and go, but the underlying inflammation usually persists. Episodes of asthma symptoms can vary in length from minutes to hours and even from days to weeks, depending on your medical treatment (see Chapter 2), the severity of your symptoms, and the character of the triggering mechanism (see Chapter 3).

- ✔ Although no cure exists for asthma, in most cases you can manage and even reverse the effects of the disease. However, poorly managed or undertreated asthma may lead to loss of airway functions and, in some cases, irreversible lung damage as a result of airway remodeling. (I explain airway remodeling in the section "How airway obstruction develops," later in this chapter.)

- ✔ Early, aggressive treatment with appropriate medication is vital to effectively managing your asthma.

Identifying asthma triggers and symptoms

A wide variety of allergens, irritants, and other factors, such as colds, flu, exercise, and drug sensitivities, can trigger asthma symptoms — what you may refer to as *asthma attacks* or *asthma episodes.* (See Chapters 3 and 4 for more about asthma triggers and how to avoid them.)

Asthma symptoms can range from decreased tolerance to exercise to feeling completely out of breath, and from persistent coughing to wheezing, chest tightness, or life-threatening respiratory distress. In many cases, a bothersome cough may be the only asthma symptom you even notice.

Experiencing asthma symptoms, whatever the intensity, means that your asthma isn't temporarily well controlled. Such symptoms may indicate that your asthma needs more effective management, as I explain in the section "Managing Your Asthma: Essential Steps," later in this chapter.

Realizing that asthma isn't in your head

Until recently, many healthcare providers and family members approached asthma as a nervous disorder, thought to be caused by anxiety and psychological stress. Doctors and researchers now know that this misconception has no basis in fact. Asthma occurs in your lungs' airways, not in your head. Although anxiety and stress can aggravate your asthma (as well as other illnesses), psychological factors don't cause your condition.

Uncovering the Many Facets of Asthma

Asthma can show up in various ways. Many asthma symptoms are caused by a complex series of events involving many types of cells and tissue that reside in your lungs. I explain this process further in the section "Asthma and Your Airways," later in this chapter.

Because such a wide range of factors can precipitate asthma symptoms, and because certain triggers can cause stronger reactions in some asthma patients than in others, doctors often classify asthma according to the triggers that instigate your symptoms. Classifying asthma in this way can help you and your doctor understand the cause of your symptoms.

Although a certain precipitating factor may predominate in many asthma cases, multiple triggers affect the majority of people with asthma. For example, most asthmatics have exercise-induced asthma (EIA), sometimes known as exercise-induced bronchospasm (EIB) — which I explain in the "Exercise-induced asthma (EIA)" section in this chapter — in addition to asthma that manifests from other triggers or precipitating factors. The next sections list the main asthma classifications that many doctors use.

Allergic asthma

Throughout the world, triggers of this common form of asthma include inhalant allergens, such as dust mites, animal dander, fungal spores, and pollens from trees, grasses, and weeds. If you suffer from allergic asthma, you may be sensitive to a combination of these allergens and probably suffer from allergic rhinitis (hay fever) and/or allergic conjunctivitis.

Develop and implement — in consultation with your doctor — an effective allergy-proofing and avoidance plan to limit your exposure to allergy triggers as part of your overall asthma management plan. (Chapters 3 and 4 explain how to avoid asthma triggers and precipitating factors.)

Depending on your degree of sensitivity and levels of exposure to inhalant allergens, your doctor may also recommend allergy testing (which an allergist usually performs) to determine what triggers your allergic asthma and whether *immunotherapy* (allergy shots) may provide an appropriate and effective treatment for your condition.

Nonallergic asthma

Irritants, such as tobacco smoke, household cleaners, soaps, perfumes and scents, glue, aerosols, smoke from wood-burning appliances or fireplaces, fumes from unvented gas, oil, or kerosene stoves, and indoor and outdoor air pollutants can also trigger asthma.

Upper respiratory tract infections, such as the common cold and flu, as well as sinusitis, nasal polyps, GERD, and aspirin sensitivity (see "Aspirin-induced and food-additive-induced asthma," later in this chapter), may also aggravate airway inflammation and trigger asthma symptoms in some people.

Occupational asthma

Current estimates are that occupational asthma, which a wide range of allergens and irritants can trigger, affects as many as 15 percent of asthma patients in the United States. The precipitating factors in occupational asthma cases often include exposure to

fumes, chemicals, gases, resins, metals, dust, insecticides, vapors, and other substances in the workplace
that can induce or aggravate airway inflammation.

Exercise-induced asthma (EIA)

Symptoms of *exercise-induced asthma* (EIA) occur to
varying degrees in a majority of asthmatics.
Exercising that involves breathing cold, dry air —
such as running outdoors in winter — may trigger EIA
symptoms more often than activities that involve
breathing warmer, humidified air, such as swimming
in a heated pool.

Certain medications can help you prevent and
control EIA symptoms (see Chapter 3) so that
you can enjoy many types of exercise and
sports activities, in spite of your condition.
You should take these medical products only
according to your doctor's advice.

Aspirin-induced and food-additive-induced asthma

A significant number of people who have both asthma
and nasal polyps may experience intensified asthma
symptoms if they take aspirin and related medications, such as over-the-counter NSAIDs and prescription NSAIDs, known as COX-2 inhibitors (celecoxib, or
Celebrex, for example).

Some asthma sufferers may also experience intensified symptoms if they ingest *sulfites* (preservatives
found in beer, wine, and many processed foods) or
tartrazine (FDC yellow dye No. 5), which is used in
many medications, foods, and vitamin products.

Asthma and Your Airways

Your airways are vital to your health. This network of bronchial tubes enables your lungs to absorb oxygen into the bloodstream and eliminate carbon dioxide — the process called *respiration,* or breathing. Most people take breathing for granted — you usually don't need to think about it, unless something interferes with this process by obstructing your airways.

The inflammatory response

In asthma, airway obstruction is most often the result of an underlying airway inflammation that leads to one or more of the following conditions (which I explain in the section "How airway obstruction develops," later in this chapter):

✔ Airway hyperresponsiveness

✔ Airway constriction

✔ Airway congestion

These airway conditions can become part of an overall, ongoing process known as the *inflammatory response.* This complex response can develop into a vicious cycle of worsening inflammation, hyperresponsiveness, constriction, and congestion, in which your airways become more sensitive and inflamed as a result of reacting to allergens, irritants, and other factors.

The ongoing, underlying airway inflammation is often so subtle that you don't notice it. Asthma symptoms are often just the tip of the iceberg. If you have asthma, the inflammation smolders away in your airways, whether or not you're actually experiencing symptoms.

Imagine if you had a rash or sunburn and only took pain relievers to deal with the discomfort, instead of staying out of the sun or treating the cause of the problem. The underlying airway inflammation in asthma is similar to having a sunburn in your bronchial tubes, as my good friend Nancy Sander, founder of the Allergy and Asthma Network/Mothers of Asthmatics (AANMA), likes to explain. If you suffer from asthma, the insides of your airways are often red and inflamed, and, as with a bad rash or sunburn, the top layer of airway tissue may peel.

If your lungs were external organs — like gills — or if your body was transparent so that you could see what happens internally, more doctors would treat asthma earlier and more aggressively because you and your doctor could easily see how the underlying disease affects you.

As I explain in the section "Testing your lungs," later in the chapter, you need to make sure that your doctor performs appropriate pulmonary (lung) function tests if you have bouts of wheezing, recurring coughs, lingering colds, or other symptoms that could indicate an underlying respiratory ailment.

How airway obstruction develops

Here's an overview of how the mechanisms of asthma interact. Although I've itemized these processes to explain them, keep in mind that they are often ongoing events that can occur simultaneously in your lungs. As you read these descriptions, take a look at Figure 1-1, which compares a normal airway with an asthmatic airway.

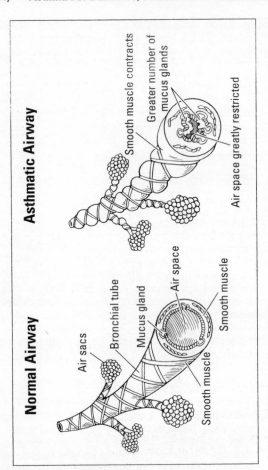

Figure 1-1: A normal airway and an asthmatic airway. Note the muscle contractions (bronchospasms) and airway inflammation.

✔ **Airway constriction:** When a trigger or precipitating factor irritates your airways, causing the
release of chemical mediators such as histamine
and leukotrienes from the mast cells of the
epithelium (the lining of the airway), the muscles around your bronchial tubes can tighten,
leading to *airway constriction*. This process
results in narrowing airways and breathing difficulty. Airway constriction can also occur in
people who don't have asthma or allergies if
they're exposed to substances that can harm
their respiratory systems, such as poisonous
gases or smoke from a burning building.

✔ **Airway hyperresponsiveness:** The underlying
airway inflammation in asthma can cause *airway
hyperresponsiveness* as the muscles around your
bronchial tubes twitch or feel ticklish. This
twitchy or ticklish feeling indicates that your
muscles overreact and tighten, causing acute
bronchoconstriction or bronchospasms even if
you're exposed only to otherwise harmless substances, such as allergens and irritants, that
rarely provoke reactions in people without
asthma and allergies (see the section
"Uncovering the Many Facets of Asthma," earlier
in the chapter).

✔ **Airway congestion:** Mucus and fluids are
released as part of the inflammatory process
and can accumulate in your airways, over-
whelming the *cilia* (tiny hairlike projections
from certain cells that sweep debris-laden
mucus through your airways) and leading to
airway congestion. This accumulation of mucus
and fluids may make you feel the urge to cough
up phlegm to relieve your chest congestion.

✔ **Airway edema:** The long-term release of inflammatory fluids in constricted, hyperresponsive,
and congested airways can lead to *airway edema*
(swelling of the airway), causing bronchial tubes

to become more rigid and further interfering with airflow. In severe cases of airway congestion and edema, a chronic buildup of mucus secretion leads to the formation of mucus plugs in the airway, which limits airflow.

✔ **Airway remodeling:** If airway inflammation is left untreated or poorly managed for many years, the constant injury to your bronchial tubes due to ongoing airway constriction, airway hyperresponsiveness, and airway congestion can lead to *airway remodeling,* as scar tissue permanently replaces your normal airway tissue. As a result of airway remodeling, airway obstruction can persist and may not respond to treatment, leading to the eventual loss of your airway function as well as potentially irreversible lung damage.

This cycle of asthma can develop gradually, over hours or even days following exposure to triggers or precipitating factors. After this cycle is set in motion, you can suffer severe and long-lasting consequences.

Diagnosing Asthma

Effectively managing your asthma begins with your doctor correctly diagnosing your condition. In order to determine whether asthma causes your respiratory symptoms, your doctor should take your medical history, perform a physical exam, test your lung functions, and perform other tests, as I explain in the following sections.

The diagnostic processes that your doctor uses are crucial because, as my friend Nancy Sander notes, asthma isn't a neat little package of symptoms that you or your doctor can easily identify and eliminate. Asthma symptoms vary widely from patient to patient. In fact, your own symptoms may change over time. Make sure your doctor establishes these key points when diagnosing your asthma:

✔ You experience episodes of airway obstruction.

✔ Your airway obstruction is at least partially reversible (and can be improved through treatment).

✔ Your symptoms result from asthma, not from other conditions that I describe in "Considering other possible diagnoses," later in this chapter.

Taking your medical history

 A careful, thorough medical history is vital in diagnosing the correct cause of your respiratory symptoms. For this reason, your doctor may ask several questions about your condition and your life. Keeping track of symptoms in a diary may help provide your doctor with details that can assist her with a proper diagnosis. Try to provide your doctor with as much information as possible about the following:

✔ The type of symptoms you experience, which may include coughing, wheezing, shortness of breath, chest tightness, and productive coughs (coughs that bring up mucus).

✔ The pattern of your symptoms. Are they *perennial* (year-round), seasonal, or perennial with seasonal worsening? Are they constant, episodic, or constant with episodic worsening?

✔ The onset of your symptoms. At what rate do your symptoms develop — rapidly or slowly? And does that rate vary?

- ✔ The duration and frequency of your symptoms and whether the type and intensity of symptoms vary at different times of day and night. Especially note whether your episodes awaken you from sleep or are more severe when you wake up in the morning.

- ✔ The impact that exercise or other physical exertion has on your symptoms.

- ✔ Your exposure to potential asthma triggers. In addition to the allergens, irritants, and precipitating factors that I list in the section "Uncovering the Many Facets of Asthma," earlier in this chapter, your doctor also needs to know about endocrine factors, such as adrenal or thyroid disease. Special considerations for women are pregnancy or changes in their menstrual cycles.

- ✔ The development of your disease, including any prior treatment and medications you've received or taken and their effectiveness. Your doctor particularly wants to know whether you presently take or have previously taken oral corticosteroids and, if so, the dosage and frequency of use.

- ✔ Your family history, especially whether parents, siblings, or close relatives suffer from asthma, allergic or nonallergic rhinitis, and other types of allergies, sinusitis, or nasal polyps.

- ✔ Your lifestyle, including whether anyone smokes in your home or the other locations where you spend time, such as work or school; and any history of substance abuse.

- ✔ Your home's characteristics, such as its age and location, type of cooling and heating system, your basement's condition, whether you have a wood-burning stove, humidifier, carpet over concrete, mold and mildew, and the types of bedding, carpeting, and furniture coverings that you use.

✔ The impact of the disease on you and your family, such as any life-threatening symptoms, emergency or urgent care treatments, or hospitalizations.

✔ The number of days you (or your child with asthma) tend to miss from school or work, the disease's economic impact, and its effect on your recreational activities.

✔ The effects of the illness on your youngster's growth, development, behavior, and extent of participation in sports if he or she has asthma.

✔ Your knowledge, perception, and beliefs about asthma and its long-term management, as well as your ability to cope with the illness.

✔ The level of support you receive from your family members and their abilities to recognize and assist you in case your symptoms suddenly worsen.

Examining your condition

A physical exam for suspected asthma usually focuses not only on your breathing passageways, but also on other characteristics and symptoms of atopic disease. The significant physical signs of asthma or allergy that your doctor looks for primarily include

✔ Chest deformity, such as an expanded or overinflated chest, as well as hunched shoulders

✔ Coughing, wheezing, shortness of breath, and other respiratory symptoms

✔ Increased nasal discharge, swelling, and the presence of nasal polyps

✔ Signs of sinus disease, such as thick or discolored nasal discharge

✔ Any allergic skin conditions, such as atopic dermatitis (eczema)

Testing your lungs

 Many people are used to routinely taking their temperature or regularly having their doctor check their pulse and blood pressure, in addition to monitoring their blood sugar and cholesterol levels on a consistent basis. However, most people aren't yet in the habit of having routine pulmonary (lung) function tests, which may be why asthma is so frequently not diagnosed at an early stage but rather after a severe episode. Objective pulmonary function tests are the most reliable means of assessing the extent to which your lung function is limited or affected.

 In order to determine whether you have airway obstruction and whether your condition is *reversible* (can improve with appropriate treatment), doctors often use a *spirometer* to measure the volume of air you exhale from your large and small airways before and 15 minutes after inhaling a short-acting beta$_2$-adrenergic bronchodilator.

 Spirometry provides many types of airflow measurements, including

- **Forced vital capacity (FVC):** The maximum volume (in liters) of air that you can exhale after taking in as deep a breath as you can.

- **Forced expiratory volume (FEV1):** The volume (in liters) of air that you're able to exhale when you breathe out with maximal effort in the first second, as forcefully as possible. Physicians determine a reduction in FEV1 as the most common indicator of airway obstruction and in patients with symptoms of asthma. This test, the most important measurement in the diagnosis and management of asthma, generally measures obstruction of the large airways, although

FEV1 can also reveal severe obstruction, if present, of the small airways. A baseline FEV1 (before using a bronchodilator) that is lower than normal but that increases by at least 12 percent 15 minutes after inhaling a short-acting bronchodilator (post-bronchodilator) allows your doctor to more conclusively establish the diagnosis of asthma.

✔ **Maximum midexpiratory flow rate (MMEF):** The middle part of your forced exhalation (in liters per second). This measurement is also referred to as the *forced expiratory flow rate between 25 and 75 percent* (FEF 25–75 percent) of FVC. A reduction in this measurement can indicate obstruction of the lungs' small airways.

Your doctor compares the values from the spirometry to the predicted normal reference values, based on your age, height, sex, and race, as established by the American Thoracic Society. The percent of the predicted normal value of your measured FEV1 is one of the major criteria your doctor uses to classify your level of asthma severity. (See Chapter 2 for information on the four levels of asthma severity.)

Doctors consider spirometry a valuable diagnostic tool for diagnosing childhood cases of asthma in children older than 4. However, for younger children, the test can be difficult, if not impossible, to perform. In those cases, your child's physician may decide that trying a peak-flow meter or another less complicated assessment process is more suitable.

Just as diabetics check their blood sugar levels with a monitoring device, you can also keep an eye on your lung functions at home with a peak-flow meter. Peak-flow meters, which are available in a variety of shapes and sizes from different manufacturers, are convenient, portable, and easy-to-use devices for monitoring *peak expiratory flow rate* (PEFR), the maximum rate of air (in liters per minute) that you can force out of your large airways, as a measurement of lung function.

This measurement isn't as accurate as spirometry, but you can easily perform it at home. Measurements of PEFR are also a vital part of long-term management of your asthma, as I explain in more depth in Chapter 2.

If spirometry indicates normal or near-normal lung functions, but asthma continues to seem the most likely cause of your symptoms, your doctor may decide that a challenge test is necessary for a more conclusive diagnosis.

Challenge tests, also called bronchoprovocation, usually involve your doctor administering small doses of inhaled methacholine or histamine to you or making you exercise under his observation. The goal is to see whether these challenges cause obstructive changes in your airways, thus provoking mild asthma symptoms. Your doctor usually measures your lung functions before and after each test.

Considering other possible diagnoses

Although asthma causes most recurring episodes of coughing, wheezing, and shortness of breath, other disorders can cause these symptoms. With infants and children, underlying problems may include

✔ An upper respiratory disease, such as allergic rhinitis or sinusitis

✔ A swallowing mechanism problem or the effects of GERD

✔ Congenital heart disease, often leading to congestive heart failure

✔ An obstruction of large airways, possibly caused by a foreign object in the trachea or main bronchi, such as a small piece of popcorn that your child may have accidentally inhaled

✔ An obstruction of large airways, possibly caused by problems of the *larynx* (the cartilaginous portion of the upper respiratory tract that contains the vocal cords) or with the vocal cords themselves

✔ An obstruction of large airways, possibly caused by benign or malignant tumors or enlarged lymph nodes

✔ An obstruction of the small airways, as a result of cystic fibrosis; abnormal development of the bronchi and lungs; or a viral infection of the *bronchioles* (small bronchi)

With adult cases, underlying problems may include

✔ Chronic bronchitis and/or emphysema, collectively referred to as *chronic obstructive pulmonary disease* (COPD)

✔ Pulmonary embolism (a blood clot, air bubble, bacteria mass, or other mass that can clog a blood vessel)

✔ Heart disease

✔ Problems of the vocal cords or the larynx (vocal cord dysfunction)

✔ Benign or malignant tumors in the airways

✔ A cough reaction due to drugs such as ACE inhibitors that you may be using to treat other conditions, such as hypertension

Classifying asthma severity

If your doctor diagnoses you with asthma based on your medical history, the physical exam, and appropriate tests, studies, and assessments, he also needs to define your condition's severity. Physicians classify asthma — whether allergic or nonallergic — according to four levels of severity.

Experts from different fields of medicine have developed these severity classifications, which provide the basis for "stepwise" management of asthma. I explain stepwise management and asthma severity levels in detail in Chapter 2.

Referring to a specialist for diagnosis

 To diagnose your condition, you or your physician should consider consulting an asthma specialist, such as an allergist or *pulmonologist* (lung doctor), when

✔ Your diagnosis is difficult to establish.

✔ Your diagnosis requires specialized testing, such as allergy testing, bronchoprovocation (see the section "Testing your lungs," earlier in this chapter), or *bronchoscopy* (an exam of the interior of your bronchi using a slender, flexible, fiber-optic bronchoscope).

✔ Your doctor advises you to consider allergy shots.

✔ Other conditions, such as sinusitis, nasal polyps, severe rhinitis, GERD, chronic bronchitis and/or emphysema (COPD), vocal cord problems, or *aspergillosis* (a fungal infection that can affect the lungs), complicate your condition or diagnosis.

- ✔ You don't seem to be doing as well as you want to be.

- ✔ You aren't able to regularly sleep through the night without being awakened by your asthma.

- ✔ You can't exercise as you want to because of asthma.

- ✔ You need to use an asthma inhaler for quick relief on a daily basis or in the middle of the night.

- ✔ You've experienced a previous emergency room visit or hospitalization for asthma or anaphylaxis.

Managing Your Asthma: Essential Steps

 If you're diagnosed with asthma, you and your doctor need to develop and implement appropriate long-term and emergency-management plans to effectively treat your condition. In my experience, motivated patients (with family members) who address their conditions through this type of thorough, individualized process almost always lead fulfilling and productive lives.

Going over the basics

Your asthma management plan requires your full participation in order to work most effectively. One of the most important ways for you to actively participate in your asthma treatment is to find out about not only the disease's complexities, but also medications, self-monitoring, allergies, triggers, and precipitating factors.

Your asthma management plan should address the following key areas:

- ✔ **Assessment and monitoring of your lung functions:** In addition to helping diagnose asthma, certain tests and assessments are vital in tracking how your condition develops and responds to prescribed treatment. See the section "Testing your lungs," earlier in the chapter, and Chapter 2 for more information.

- ✔ **Avoidance measures:** Ways of avoiding and controlling your exposure to asthma triggers and precipitating factors.

- ✔ **Medication:** Using appropriate medication to prevent symptoms if you're exposed to allergens, irritants, and other asthma triggers. Depending on the severity of your symptoms, you may need to use long-term pharmacotherapy or short-term pharmacotherapy.

  Long-term pharmacotherapy involves using medications to prevent symptoms by treating the underlying airway inflammation, congestion, constriction, and hyperresponsiveness.

  Short-term pharmacotherapy involves using fast-acting rescue medications when your condition suddenly deteriorates.

- ✔ **Knowing when an attack is serious:** This knowledge is based on frequency of rescue inhaler use, decrease in peak-flow values, and increased nighttime awakenings.

- ✔ **Determining what to do if you have a serious attack:** You should know how to adjust your medication in response to a worsening of symptoms and when to call for medical help if your condition continues to deteriorate.

- ✔ **An ongoing process of education for you and your family about asthma:** This process can involve information and resources that your doctor, clinic staff, and patient support groups provide or recommend, as well as books, newsletters, videos, and other helpful materials that you and your family gather.

Determining your asthma therapy goals

Your asthma management plan should be results-oriented. I advise developing an overall goal, in consultation with your doctor, that aims for the highest attainable improvement of lung functions and enables you to maintain near-normal levels of exercise and other physical activities.

Other results that you should expect from asthma therapy include

- ✔ Preventing chronic and troublesome symptoms of asthma, such as coughing, shortness of breath, wheezing (especially upon awakening in the morning), and episodes that disturb your sleep at night
- ✔ Preventing recurring aggravation of symptoms
- ✔ Minimizing the need for emergency care and hospitalization
- ✔ Providing the most effective medication therapy that results in minimal or no adverse side effects

Based on the previous goals, if you feel that your doctor isn't providing adequate and effective treatment for your condition, consult an asthma specialist, such as an allergist or pulmonologist. Too often, people receive referrals only after their symptoms have gotten out of control. In my experience, after patients receive appropriate care for their asthma and understand that, in most cases, their asthma management goals are clearly achievable, they usually lead normal lives and don't tolerate going back to being frequently ill with asthma attacks.

You or your physician may also want to consider consulting an asthma specialist if

- ✔ You've suffered a life-threatening asthma attack.

- ✔ You're not meeting the goals of your asthma therapy.

- ✔ You require more education and guidance on possible treatment complications, the avoidance and control of triggers and precipitating factors, and your asthma management program.

- ✔ You have severe persistent asthma that requires constant daily use of preventive medications and frequent use of short-acting inhaled beta$_2$-adrenergic (beta$_2$-agonist) bronchodilators.

- ✔ Your condition requires continuous use of oral corticosteroids, high-dose inhaled corticosteroids, or more than two bursts of oral corticosteroids within one year.

- ✔ You have a child under age 3 who has moderate persistent or severe persistent asthma (see Chapter 2) and requires constant use of preventive medication and frequent use of short-acting inhaled beta$_2$-adrenergic bronchodilators.

- ✔ You care for a person with asthma who experiences significant psychological, emotional, or family problems that interfere with or prevent that person from following an appropriate asthma management plan. Such experiences can lead to worsening asthma symptoms, which pose a threat to the patient's health. In this event, have him or her undergo an evaluation by a mental health professional.

Handling emergencies

 In addition to instructing you on how to monitor your symptoms to recognize early warning signs of a worsening condition, your doctor should also

✔ Give you a written action plan that you can follow in case your condition deteriorates. Children with asthma need a plan that they can use at school, daycare, or summer camp. Your written action plan must clearly instruct you on how to adjust your medications in response to particular signs, symptoms, and PEFR levels, as well as tell you when to call for medical help.

✔ Instruct you to seek medical help early if your episode is severe, if medication doesn't provide rapid, sustained improvement, or if your condition continues to deteriorate.

✔ Advise you to keep on hand appropriate medications, peak-flow meters, and inhalant devices, such as nebulizers, to treat severe episodes at home if you suffer from moderate-to-severe persistent asthma or have a history of severe asthma attacks.

✔ Warn you against trying to manage severe episodes with home remedies, such as drinking large amounts of water; breathing steam or moist air (from a hot shower); taking OTC medications such as antihistamines, cold and flu remedies, and pain relievers; or using OTC bronchodilators. Although these types of inhalers can sometimes provide temporary relief of airway constriction, they certainly aren't the preferable approach when appropriate medical care is required for treating acute asthma emergencies.

Chapter 2

The Basics of Managing Asthma Long-Term

. . . .

In This Chapter

▶ Understanding long-term management

▶ Identifying the four levels of severity

▶ Taking the stepwise approach to treatment

▶ Evaluating your lungs

▶ Figuring out self-management

▶ Enhancing your life and overall health

. . . .

*R*ather than letting your asthma control you, the key to controlling your asthma is to treat it on a consistent and preventive basis. Doing so means managing your asthma for the long term, rather than dealing with symptoms and episodes only temporarily.

Developing and sticking to a long-term asthma management strategy is a priceless investment in your overall health and quality of life, especially if you have persistent asthma. The point is to address the root cause of your symptoms — the underlying airway inflammation that characterizes asthma.

In most cases, I find that after patients realize how much better they can feel by effectively managing their asthma long-term, they don't put up with going back to the ineffective, short-term, crisis-management ways of dealing with their disease.

Seeing What a Long-Term Management Plan Includes

A comprehensive long-term management plan for persistent asthma should include the following:

- ✔ Objective testing and monitoring of your lung functions to diagnose your condition and continuously assess the effectiveness of your treatment (see Chapter 1 and "Assessing Your Lungs" and "Taking Stock of Your Condition," later in this chapter, for details).

- ✔ Avoiding and controlling exposures to asthma triggers and precipitating factors (see Chapters 3 and 4).

- ✔ Developing a safe and effective pharmacotherapy program that results in minimal or no adverse side effects. The program includes taking appropriate long-term preventive medications on a routine basis to control your asthma and using appropriate short-term, quick-relief rescue medications if your symptoms suddenly get worse (see Chapter 5).

- ✔ Initiating pharmacotherapy with a *stepwise* (step-up or step-down) approach. (See "Using the Stepwise Approach," later in this chapter.)

- ✔ Consulting with an asthma specialist, such as an allergist or *pulmonologist* (lung doctor), when advisable (see Chapter 1).

✔ Tailoring your asthma management plan to your specific circumstances and condition, and continuing education for you and your family about asthma (see "Understanding Self-Management," later in this chapter).

Focusing on the Four Levels of Asthma Severity

Experts from different fields of medicine have classified the severity of asthma — whether allergic or nonallergic — into four levels. These asthma severity levels provide the basis for the stepwise management of the disease.

Bear in mind that these levels of severity aren't permanent or static. Asthma is a condition that can change throughout your life. The primary goal of the stepwise approach that I describe in this chapter is to get your asthma to the lowest classification possible. Therefore, effectively treating your condition is crucial: Otherwise, your asthma severity may move up the classification scale to the point where you can potentially suffer from severe, relentless symptoms that adversely affect your quality of life.

As described in the National Institutes of Health (NIH) Guidelines for the Diagnosis and Management of Asthma, the four levels of asthma severity are

✔ **Mild intermittent.** Symptoms occur no more than twice a week during the day and no more than twice a month at night. Lung-function testing (see Chapter 1) shows 80 percent or greater of the predicted normal value, compared to reference values based on your age, height, sex, and race, as established by the American Thoracic Society. In addition, your peak expiratory flow rate (PEFR; see Chapter 1) shouldn't vary by more than 20 percent during episodes and from the morning to the evening. Between episodes, you may be *asymptomatic* (not have noticeable symptoms), and your PEFR should be normal. If your asthma is at this level, a worsening of symptoms is usually brief, lasting a few hours to a few days, with variations of intensity.

✔ **Mild persistent.** Symptoms occur more than twice a week during the day, but less than once a day, and more than twice a month, at night. Lung-function testing shows 80 percent or greater of the predicted normal value. Your PEFR may vary between 20 and 30 percent. If your asthma is at this level of severity, then worsening of symptoms can begin to affect your activities.

✔ **Moderate persistent.** Symptoms occur daily and more than once a week at night, requiring daily use of a short-acting bronchodilator. Lung-function testing shows a 60- to 80-percent range of the normal predicted value. Your PEFR can vary more than 30 percent. Symptoms can worsen at least twice a week, with episodes lasting for days and affecting your activities.

✔ **Severe persistent.** Symptoms occur continuously during the day and frequently at night, limiting physical activity. Lung-function testing is 60 percent or less of the normal predicted value. Your PEFR may vary more than 30 percent, and frequent aggravations of your condition can develop.

When diagnosing your condition, your doctor should identify your asthma's severity level. Check to see which of the severity levels your condition most resembles, based on the definitions that I list in this section. Your own symptoms and lung functions may not always fit neatly into one of these particular severity levels. Your doctor, therefore, should evaluate your individual condition and develop a treatment plan for you based on the specific characteristics of your asthma. Based on symptom criteria and the results of lung-function testing, the vast majority of asthma patients have some form of persistent asthma — mild, moderate, or severe — requiring long-term control therapy.

 If the symptoms you're experiencing seem to indicate that you have persistent asthma, I strongly advise having your lung functions evaluated by *spirometry* if you haven't already done so (see "Assessing Your Lungs," later in this chapter). For a spirometry evaluation, you may need to ask your doctor for a referral to an asthma specialist, such as an allergist or pulmonologist, because in many cases, primary care physicians don't have easy access to office spirometers.

Using the Stepwise Approach

Asthma severity levels are steps in the staircase to controlling asthma, as shown in Figure 2-1. The basic concept of stepwise management is to initially prescribe long-term and quick-relief medications, based on the severity level that's one step higher than the severity level you're experiencing. By using this approach, your doctor can usually help you gain rapid control over your symptoms. After your condition has been under control for a month (in most cases), your physician can reduce the level of your medications by one level *(step down)*.

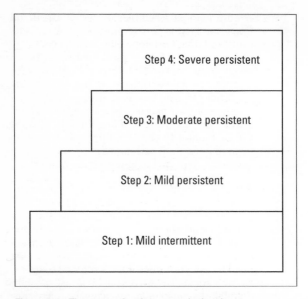

Figure 2-1: The steps of asthma severity levels.

  Using the stepwise approach to asthma management means that you *step up* your medication
therapy to gain control, and then *step down* your
medical treatment to maintain control. Like
waltzing, after you and your doctor master the
steps, you can move around life's dance floor
with the ease and grace of Fred Astaire or
Ginger Rogers. Regular monitoring of your PEFR,
and follow-up visits with your doctor are vital to
ensuring that you stay in step.

The information in the following list is based on the
NIH Guidelines for the Diagnosis and Management of
Asthma in adults and children older than 5. Please

remember that these are guidelines. Your doctor should always evaluate your own specific condition and prescribe individualized treatment accordingly.

✔ **Step 1: Mild intermittent.** No daily medication is needed for long-term control.

✔ **Step 2: Mild persistent.** One daily medication for long-term control: anti-inflammatory medication, either inhaled corticosteroid (low dose) or mast cell stabilizers, such as cromolyn or nedocromil. Your doctor may also consider anti-leukotriene modifiers such as zafirlukast and montelukast, or a methylxanthine product such as sustained-release theophylline as an alternative treatment, but not as preferred therapy.

✔ **Step 3: Moderate persistent.** Daily medication for long-term control: anti-inflammatory medication, inhaled corticosteroid (medium dose), or inhaled corticosteroid (low to medium dose), adding a long-acting bronchodilator, especially for nighttime symptoms — either long-acting inhaled beta$_2$-adrenergics, sustained release theophylline, or long-acting beta$_2$-adrenergic tablets.

If needed: anti-inflammatory medication, inhaled corticosteroid (medium-high dose), and long-acting bronchodilator, especially for nighttime symptoms — either long-acting inhaled beta$_2$-adrenergics, sustained release theophylline, or long-acting beta$_2$-adrenergic tablets.

✔ **Step 4: Severe persistent.** Daily medication for long-term control: anti-inflammatory medication, inhaled corticosteroid (high dose), and long-acting bronchodilator — either long-acting inhaled beta$_2$-adrenergics, sustained release theophylline, or long-acting beta$_2$-adrenergic tablets; and if required, long-term use of corticosteroid tablets or syrup.

For quick relief at any step, use a short-acting bron-chodilator: inhaled beta$_2$-adrenergics as needed for symptoms. Intensity of treatment may vary depending on the severity of your symptoms. (If you're using a short-acting inhaled beta$_2$-adrenergic more than twice a week, you may need additional long-term control therapy. Consult your doctor in this case.)

If your asthma severity is at Step 3 or Step 4, consult an asthma specialist, such as an allergist or pulmonologist (lung doctor), to achieve better control of your condition.

Stepping down

If you're on long-term maintenance control at any level, your doctor should review your treatment every one to six months. A gradual stepwise reduction in treatment may be possible after your symptoms are under good control, meaning that you feel good, have maintained improved lung function, and experience no asthma symptoms.

The goal of the stepwise approach is to use early and aggressive treatment to gain rapid control over your asthma symptoms, thus allowing your doctor to reduce your medication to the lowest level required to maintain control of your condition.

Stepping up

If you find yourself frequently resorting to your quick-relief medications, your symptoms aren't under control, and your doctor should consider increasing your treatment by one step. In assessing whether to step up your therapy, your doctor will probably evaluate the following aspects of your current treatment step:

✔ Your inhaler technique. (See "Evaluating your inhaler technique," later in this chapter.)

✔ Your level of adherence in taking the medications that your doctor prescribes. Taking your prescriptions as your doctor instructs is vital. If you're having trouble with a product (because of potential side effects) or you don't understand your doctor's instructions, tell your physician so he can take appropriate measures. (See Chapter 5 for more about medication.)

✔ Your exposure level to asthma triggers, such as allergens and irritants, and precipitating factors, such as viral infections and other medical conditions. Control your exposure to asthma triggers and precipitating factors as much as possible, no matter what step of treatment you're receiving. (See Chapters 3 and 4 for info on controlling triggers and avoiding allergens.)

Make sure that your asthma management plan clearly explains at what point you should contact your physician if your symptoms worsen.

Treating severe episodes

Your doctor may consider prescribing a rescue course of oral corticosteroids at any step if you suddenly experience a severe asthma episode and your condition abruptly deteriorates. (Chapter 5 provides more information on oral corticosteroids.)

In some cases, severe episodes can occur even if your asthma is classified as intermittent. In many instances, patients with intermittent asthma may experience severe and potentially life-threatening episodes, often because of upper respiratory viral infections (such as the flu or colds), even though these patients may otherwise have long periods of normal or near-normal lung functions and few clinically perceptible asthma symptoms.

Assessing Your Lungs

Objective measurements of your lung functions are essential for monitoring your asthma's severity. Just as you check the oil level in your car on a regular basis (instead of waiting for the flashing red warning light), you and your doctor should also regularly check your airways to determine whether you're at the right step of asthma medication. In addition to recording your asthma symptoms in a daily symptom diary (see "Keeping symptom records," later in this chapter), you should also obtain objective measurements of lung functions with spirometry and peak-flow monitoring.

Spirometry

A *spirometer* is a sophisticated machine that your doctor or asthma specialist, such as an allergist or pulmonologist, uses for measuring airflow from your large and small airways before and 15 minutes after you've inhaled from a short-acting bronchodilator. The spirometer helps your asthma specialist diagnose whether you have asthma and also allows your physician to follow your asthma's clinical course.

For adults and children older than age 4 or 5, spirometry currently provides the most accurate way of determining whether airway obstruction exists and whether it's reversible. For information on other types of lung-function tests your doctor may recommend, and to find out more about diagnosing asthma in children under age 4, see Chapter 1.

Peak-flow monitoring

Peak-flow meters allow you to keep an eye on your lung functions at home. The readings from this handy tool can be vital in diagnosing asthma and its severity, and can also help your doctor prescribe medications and monitor your treatment's effectiveness. Peak-flow monitoring can also provide important early warning signs that an asthma episode is approaching.

Children older than 4 or 5 who have asthma generally can also use this small, hand-held device to measure their own PEFR. If your kids constantly question your judgment (as mine do about almost everything), using a peak-flow meter can help youngsters understand when their condition may require them to limit their activities. If your child understands that the PEFR — not just you or your doctor — is advising him or her not to go to soccer practice on that particular day because of worsening asthma symptoms and a resulting PEFR reduction, you may have more success in helping to control your child's asthma.

Consider these basic instructions and tips for using most types of peak-flow meters (several different makes and models are currently available). Remember, however, to follow the instructions that come with your specific device. Ask your doctor for specific advice on the most effective way you can use your peak-flow meter to assess your condition.

Generally, you use a peak-flow meter by following these steps:

1. **Move the sliding indicator at the base of the peak-flow meter to zero.**

2. **Stand up and take a deep breath to fully inflate your lungs.**

3. **Put the mouthpiece of the peak-flow meter into your mouth and close your lips tightly around it.**

4. **Blow as hard and as fast as possible, like you're blowing out the candles on your birthday cake.**

5. **Read the dial where the red indicator stopped. The number opposite the indicator is your peak-flow rate.**

6. **Reset the indicator to zero and repeat the process twice more.**

7. **Record the highest number that you reach.**

Your personal best peak-flow number is a measurement that reflects the highest number you can expect to achieve over a two- to three-week period after a course of aggressive treatment has produced good control of your asthma symptoms. Your best number is usually the result of step-up therapy.

 To determine your personal best peak-flow number, take two peak-flow readings a day during an entire week when you're doing well, and record the best result. Take one reading prior to taking medication in the morning and another reading between noon and 2 p.m. after taking an inhaled short-acting bronchodilator. Compare your personal best peak-flow number with the measurement that your physician predicts, which is based on national studies for children or adults of particular heights, sexes, and ages. This number can help you determine how your measurements compare with the norm. When your asthma is well controlled, your PEFR should consistently read between 80 and 100 percent of your personal best.

 If your peak-flow measurements fall below 80 percent, early and aggressive intervention with medications and strict avoidance of potential asthma triggers may be necessary to prevent worsening symptoms. Ignoring a declining peak-flow reading can lead to serious symptoms and may result in the need for emergency treatment.

The peak-flow zone system involves green, yellow, and red areas, which are similar to a traffic signal. Using your peak-flow meter on a regular basis enables you and your doctor to treat symptoms before your condition deteriorates further.

You or your doctor may want to place small pieces of colored tape next to the actual numbers on your peak-flow meter, corresponding with the green, yellow, and red zones that your doctor provides as a graph on your written asthma peak-flow diary. (See "Keeping symptom records," later in the chapter, for more about asthma diaries.)

Table 2-1 explains how to read peak-flow color zones.

Table 2-1	The Peak-Flow Color Zone System	
Zone	*Meaning*	*Points to Consider*
Green zone	Readings in this area are *safe.*	When your reading falls into the green zone, you've achieved 80 to 100 percent of your personal best peak flow. No asthma symptoms are present, and your treatment plan is controlling your asthma. If your readings consistently remain in the green zone, you and your doctor may consider reducing daily medications.

(continued)

Table 2-1 *(continued)*

Zone	Meaning	Points to Consider
Yellow zone	Readings in this area indicate *caution.*	When your readings fall into the yellow zone, you're achieving only 50 to 80 percent of your personal best peak flow. An asthma attack may be present, and your symptoms may worsen. You may need to step up your medication temporarily.
Red zone	Readings in this area mean *medical alert.*	Readings in the red zone mean that you've fallen below 50 percent of your personal best peak flow. These readings often signal the start of a moderate to severe asthma attack.

 If your readings are often in the yellow zone, even after taking the appropriate quick-relief medication that your asthma management plan specifies, contact your doctor. If your readings are in the red zone, use your quick-relief bronchodilator and anti-inflammatory medications immediately (based on your specific and individualized asthma management plan), and contact your doctor if your PEFR doesn't immediately return to and remain in the yellow or green zone.

Taking Stock of Your Condition

In addition to obtaining an objective measurement of
your lung function with measuring devices, another
important aspect of controlling your asthma is keeping track of a variety of other indicators. Your most
valuable tracking device is usually a daily symptom
diary. In fact, you should develop a rating system (in
consultation with your doctor) for your diary that
assesses your symptoms on a scale of 0 to 3, ranging
from no symptoms to severe symptoms.

Keeping symptom records

Besides serving as a record of your PEFR readings, your daily symptom diary should monitor
and record the following:

✔ Your signs and symptoms, as well as their
severity

✔ Any coughing that you experience

✔ Any incidence of wheezing

✔ Nasal congestion

✔ Disturbances in your sleep, such as coughing
and/or wheezing that awaken you

✔ Any symptoms that affect your ability to function normally or reduce normal activities

✔ Any time you miss school or work because of
symptoms

✔ Frequency of use of your short-acting beta$_2$-
adrenergic bronchodilator (rescue medication)

Tracking serious symptoms

 Your daily symptom diary is also the place to monitor occurrences of symptoms severe enough to make you seek unscheduled office visits, after-hours treatments, emergency room visits, and hospitalizations. Therefore, you also want to note the date and kind of treatment that you seek.

Be sure to record the following serious symptoms:

- ✔ Breathlessness or panting while at rest
- ✔ The need to remain in an upright position in order to breathe
- ✔ Difficulty speaking
- ✔ Agitation or confusion
- ✔ An increased breathing rate of more than 30 breaths per minute
- ✔ Loud wheezing while inhaling and/or exhaling
- ✔ An elevated pulse rate of more than 120 heartbeats per minute

Furthermore, record exposures to triggers and/or precipitating factors (see Chapters 3 and 4) that may have caused asthma flare-ups, including

- ✔ Irritants, such as chemicals or cigarette or fireplace smoke
- ✔ Allergens, such as plant pollen, household dust, molds, and animal fur
- ✔ Air pollution
- ✔ Exercise
- ✔ Sudden changes in the weather, particularly cold temperatures and chilly winds

✔ Reactions to beta-blockers (such as Inderal or Timoptic), aspirin, and related products, including nonsteroidal anti-inflammatory drugs (NSAIDs) and food additives — particularly sulfites

✔ Other medical conditions, such as upper respiratory viral infections (colds and flu), gastroesophageal reflux disease (GERD), and sinusitis

Monitoring your medication use

Recording all the side effects that you experience when taking your prescribed medication is also important. Various asthma medications include many levels of side effects that a person can potentially experience. However, in most cases, patients who understand their asthma management plan and take their medications according to instructions have few, if any, adverse side effects. See Chapter 5 for more about medication.

I need to emphasize how important it is to know and remember the names of your medications, especially if you're an older adult with multiple prescriptions. Patients telling me they're using a "white inhaler" or taking a "yellow pill" aren't providing the most helpful information in my quest to provide the best care possible and prevent potential adverse drug interactions with medications prescribed by another physician.

Evaluating your inhaler technique

Your doctor should show you the correct way to use your inhaler and have you demonstrate your inhaler technique at each office visit. In the best of cases when using inhalers, only 10 to 20 percent of the topical inhaled drug gets into the areas of your lungs where it can really do some good. Because such small amounts of inhaler medications actually reach the airways of your lungs, understanding how to use your inhaler properly is vital to your treatment. Improper inhaler use is often the reason why some patients have difficulty controlling their asthma symptoms.

Understanding Self-Management

It takes two (at least) to treat asthma. You and your physician (as well as your other healthcare providers) are partners in controlling your asthma. Other members of your partnership can include nurses, pharmacists, and other health professionals who treat you or assist you in understanding and finding out more about effectively managing your condition.

If you have asthma, your family also — in a sense — has asthma. Asthma isn't contagious; rather, your family also has the condition because you all may need to deal with the various issues associated with your medical condition's treatment. In fact, studies show that family support can be a major positive factor in the success of any asthma treatment plan. Particularly important to your asthma treatment is making sure that the people you live with (as well as co-workers, fellow students, or anyone you're around much of the time) help you reduce your exposure to asthma triggers and to precipitating factors. I explain the most common triggers and precipitating factors to avoid in Chapter 3.

If your child has asthma, you should be a partner with your child's doctor and other medical professionals in the management of your child's condition.

Working with your doctor

Participate in developing treatment goals with your doctor. Make sure that you understand how your asthma management plan works and that you can openly communicate with your doctor about the effects and results of your treatment.

Making sure that your plan is tailored to your specific, individualized needs, as well as your family's, is also very important. Doing so can include taking into account any cultural beliefs and practices that can have an impact on your perception of asthma and of medication therapy. Openly discuss any such issues with your physician, so that together, you can develop an approach to asthma management that empowers you to take control of your condition. Ensuring that your plan is tailored to fit you and your family results in a more motivated patient, which almost always means a healthier individual.

Evaluating for the long term

Successfully managing your asthma also means constantly assessing your asthma management plan to determine whether it provides you with the means to achieve your asthma management goals.

Always keep in mind that asthma is a variable, complex, multifaceted condition. Just as many other aspects of your life can change and vary over time, your asthma may also manifest in different ways throughout your life. Remember: Your goal is lifetime management of your condition.

Being an expert about your asthma

The education process concerning asthma and its treatment should begin as soon as you're diagnosed. I believe that your doctor should make sure that you have a thorough understanding of all aspects of your condition. Ignorance is not bliss when it comes to managing your asthma effectively. Your process of education should include factors such as the following:

✔ Knowing the basic facts about asthma.

✔ Understanding the level of your asthma severity, how it affects you, and advisable treatment methods.

✔ Teaching you all the elements of asthma self-management, including basic facts about the disease and your specific condition, proper use of various inhalers and nebulizers, self-monitoring skills, and effective ways of avoiding triggers and allergy-proofing your home.

✔ Developing a written individualized daily and emergency self-management plan with your input (see Chapter 1).

✔ Determining the level of support you receive from family and friends in treating your asthma. It's also important for your doctor to help you identify an asthma partner from among your family members, relatives, or friends. This person should find out how asthma affects you and should understand your asthma management plan so that he or she can provide assistance (if necessary) if your condition suddenly worsens. I advise including your asthma partner in doctor visits when appropriate.

✔ Asking your doctor and/or other members of your asthma management team for guidance in setting priorities when implementing your asthma management plan. If you need to make environmental changes in your life, such as allergy-proofing your home (which may include relocating a pet, taking up the carpets, installing air filtration devices, and many other steps that I explain in Chapter 3), you may want advice on which steps you need to take soonest and which steps can wait.

Improving Your Quality of Life

Taking asthma medication doesn't mean that you can afford to ignore other aspects of your health. Effectively managing your asthma for the long term also requires being healthy overall. The better you take care of yourself, the more success you'll have in treating your asthma and living a full, normal life.

Consider these important, common-sense guidelines when developing an asthma management plan:

- ✔ **Eating right.** A healthy, well-balanced diet is especially important for people who have asthma. Include fresh fruits, meats, fish, grains, and vegetables in your diet.

- ✔ **Sleeping well.** If you experience symptoms during the night that disturb your sleep, tell your doctor. These types of symptoms should be treated, and they may indicate that you're susceptible to precipitating factors, such as GERD, or asthma triggers such as dust mites in your bedroom (see Chapter 3).

- ✔ **Staying fit.** When patients are in good physical condition, their asthma is often easier to control. You don't have to sit on life's sidelines just because you have asthma. Your doctor can prescribe medications that you can take preventively to control symptoms of EIA (exercise-induced asthma), thus enabling you to enjoy many types of exercise and sports activities in spite of your asthma. (Chapter 3 has details on products for controlling EIA.)

✔ **Reducing stress.** By effectively controlling your asthma, you'll feel less anxious about your condition, thus reducing your overall levels of stress and further helping you manage your asthma.

Expecting the Best

With effective, appropriate care from your doctor and your own motivated participation as a patient, your asthma management plan can enable you to lead a full and active life. However, if properly following your asthma management plan still doesn't allow you to participate fully in the activities and pursuits that matter to you, openly communicate this information to your physician so that she can adjust your plan and maximize the effectiveness of your treatment.

If, as sometimes happens, your doctor deals only with your asthma symptoms — instead of initiating the type of long-term approach that I discuss in this chapter — you may want to consider requesting a referral to an asthma specialist. Expect to effectively control your asthma, and your doctor should certainly help you achieve this goal.

Chapter 3

Understanding Asthma Triggers

. . . .

In This Chapter

▷ Identifying what's triggering your asthma

▷ Avoiding inhalant allergens

▷ Focusing on triggers in your home

▷ Recognizing triggers in your workplace

▷ Steering clear of food and drug triggers

▷ Dealing with other conditions that can aggravate asthma

. . . .

*W*ater covers two-thirds of the world's surface. If you have asthma, it may seem at times that the rest of the planet consists of nothing but asthma triggers. Throughout the world and in virtually every aspect of people's everyday lives, countless precipitating factors — allergens, irritants, or other medical conditions — can induce asthma symptoms.

Avoiding or limiting your exposure to these precipitating factors is vital for managing your condition. Avoiding asthma triggers can help you experience fewer respiratory symptoms and potentially allow you to reduce your need for medication, especially rescue drugs such as short-acting $beta_2$-adrenergic ($beta_2$-agonist) bronchodilators. (See Chapter 5 for details.)

Although certain triggers frequently dominate each individual's asthma, controlling your condition often requires dealing with a host of precipitating factors — an especially common situation if you have allergic asthma. Allergic asthma is usually associated with *allergic rhinitis* (hay fever) and/or allergic conjunctivitis (see Chapter 1 for details).

If the prospect of dealing with a world full of asthma triggers seems daunting, don't despair. In this chapter, I provide information and tips, based on extensive experience and the latest research findings, that can help you — in consultation with your doctor — implement practical and effective measures for avoiding or reducing exposure to triggers.

Recognizing What Triggers Your Asthma

One of the most important steps you need to take to effectively manage your asthma is to identify what triggers the symptoms. Triggers may include

- ✔ Inhalant allergens, including animal danders, dust mite and cockroach allergens, some mold spores, and certain airborne pollens of grasses, weeds, and trees (see Chapter 4).

- ✔ Occupational irritants and allergens, found primarily in the workplace, that induce occupational asthma or aggravate an already existing form of the disease.

✔ Other irritants that you inhale, such as tobacco smoke, household products, and indoor and outdoor air pollution.

✔ Nonallergic triggers, including exercise and physical stimuli such as variations in air temperature and humidity levels.

✔ Other medical conditions, including rhinitis, sinusitis, gastroesophageal reflux disease (GERD), and viral infections; sensitivities to aspirin, beta-blockers, and other drugs; and sensitivities to food additives.

✔ Emotional activities, such as crying, laughing, or even yelling. Although emotions aren't the direct triggers of asthma symptoms, activities associated with emotions (happy or sad) can induce coughing or wheezing in people with pre-existing hyperreactive airways, as well as in individuals who don't have asthma but who may suffer from other respiratory disorders.

Evaluating triggers

In order to determine what triggers your asthma symptoms and your sensitivity levels to those triggers, your doctor should take a thorough medical history. Keeping an asthma diary (see Chapter 2) can assist in your doctor's assessment by providing details of your symptoms and your exposures to potential triggers. Prepare to give your doctor specific information about the respiratory symptoms that you experience.

Testing for allergic triggers

Many asthma patients experience *perennial* (year-round) symptoms that worsen during particular seasons. Because a range of triggers can contribute to perennial asthma episodes, provide your doctor with a record of the seasonal patterns of your symptoms. Your record contains clues to help your doctor narrow down the factors that affect your condition.

If you have persistent asthma (see Chapter 2) with year-round symptoms that occur primarily indoors, allergy testing can help your doctor identify several triggers, such as dust mites, that may be affecting you.

Nocturnal or *nighttime asthma,* which often shows up as a nighttime cough, wheezing, and/or shortness of breath that disturbs your sleep and may require you to use your short-acting adrenergic bronchodilator (see Chapter 5), can often be severe. Allergens in your bedroom, postnasal drip from allergic rhinitis, or chronic sinus problems (such as sinusitis) often trigger this condition. Other mechanisms that can trigger nocturnal asthma include

- ✔ GERD

- ✔ Airway cooling and drying

- ✔ Increased bronchial airway hyperreactivity

- ✔ A delayed reaction (known as a *late-phase reaction*) to allergens that you've been exposed to previously during the day

The *circadian rhythm* (also known as *diurnal variation*), which is your body's internal clock, may also affect your asthma, making you more susceptible to symptoms in the early morning hours (around 3 to 5 a.m.). During the late evening and early morning hours, a decrease in plasma levels of *adrenal gland* (glands above your kidneys) *hormones,* such as *cortisol,* a hormone produced by the *cortex* (outer layer) of the adrenal gland, normally occurs. At the same time, a decrease in plasma epinephrine and an increase in plasma histamine also occur.

Controlling Inhalant Allergens

Inhalant allergen triggers, also known as *aeroallergens,* are probably the most familiar asthma precipitants because they're also associated with allergic rhinitis and similar conditions. If you have allergic asthma, reducing your exposure to inhalant allergens is the first and most important step to take — in consultation with your doctor — to manage your condition.

The following list details the most common inhalant allergens to look out for (see Chapter 4 for details on minimizing your exposure to these allergens):

- ✔ Animal allergens
- ✔ Dust mites
- ✔ Cockroaches (for information on how to avoid cockroach allergens, see the "Curbing cockroach contamination" sidebar in this chapter)
- ✔ Mold
- ✔ Pollen

Clearing the Air at Home

Indoor environments at home, work, and school and in cars as well as other enclosed means of transportation can often provide more significant sources of asthma triggers than the outdoors, because most enclosures concentrate irritants and allergens. Therefore, you should seriously consider the effects of indoor air pollution because it can induce or aggravate asthma.

Curbing cockroach contamination

Control cockroach allergens in your home by

- ✔ Exterminating cockroach infestations. During the fumigation process, stay out of your home, and allow it to air out for several hours before re-entering. (This advice applies to anyone, regardless of whether or not you have asthma.)

- ✔ Cleaning your home thoroughly after extermination.

- ✔ Setting roach traps.

- ✔ Sealing any cracks or other conduits into your home to prevent reinfestation.

- ✔ Keeping your kitchen clean by washing dishes and cookware promptly and by emptying garbage and recycling containers (including old newspapers) often, and avoid leaving food out.

Household irritants

 The most significant irritant triggers of asthma in many households are

- ✔ Tobacco smoke (see the next section)
- ✔ Fumes and scents from household cleaners, soaps, perfumes, glues, and aerosols
- ✔ Smoke from wood-burning appliances or fireplaces
- ✔ Fumes from unvented gas, oil, or kerosene stoves

Other sources of indoor air pollution include pollens and mold spores that get inside, especially on windy days when windows and doors are open. These materials can also infiltrate your home via your clothing and hair. In fact, if you have allergic asthma, you may wake up congested and wheezing in the morning because allergenic materials find their way into your house easily. (The pollen or mold spores in your hair probably wound up on your pillow, so you spent the night breathing them into your lungs.)

No smoking, please

As far as truly irritating irritants go, tobacco smoke is the No.1 indoor air pollutant. Secondhand smoke has been associated with an increase in the following adverse effects: persistent wheezing associated with asthma, hospital admissions for respiratory infections, earlier onset of respiratory allergies, decreased lung function, and even increased incidence of *otitis media with effusion* (inflammation of the middle ear).

Tobacco smoke frequently precipitates asthma symptoms in children. Numerous studies show that parental smoking, especially by the mother, is a major risk factor in the development of asthma in infants, who are exposed to the smoke during the first few months of life. Therefore, don't smoke, and make sure that those people around you don't smoke, especially if you have children.

Filters and air-cleaning devices

The quality of the air you breathe indoors largely depends on the condition of your heating, ventilation, and air-conditioning (HVAC) system, as well as the air and particles that circulate throughout it.

If you're exposed to airborne allergens and irritants, such as animal dander, mold spores, pollen, and tobacco smoke, consider using air filters on your HVAC ducts to reduce the level of allergy and asthma triggers circulating through your home. Keep in mind, however, that these filters don't remove substances that have already settled in bedding, carpeting, and furniture — especially dust mite allergens. Dust mite allergens are generally larger than other airborne allergens and irritants, and they usually fall from the air within a few minutes after being stirred up in dust or air currents.

The two types of air filtration systems often recommended by doctors for reducing indoor levels of airborne allergens and irritants are

- ✔ **High Efficiency Particulate Arrester (HEPA):** These filters are designed to absorb and contain 99.97 percent of all particles larger than 0.3 microns (one-three hundredth the width of a human hair). If the unit truly operates at that level, only 3 out of 10,000 particles get into your indoor environment. Vacuum cleaners and air purifiers with HEPA and ULPA filters (see the next bullet for more information) can play a vital part in allergy-proofing your home.

- ✔ **Ultra Low Penetration Air (ULPA):** This system filters more thoroughly than the HEPA process and is designed to absorb and contain 99.99 percent of all particles larger than 0.12 microns.

If your home doesn't have a central HVAC system, you can purchase stand-alone HEPA and ULPA air cleaners for use in individual rooms.

Vacuum cleaning is also vital for reducing your exposure to allergens and irritants at home. However, many standard vacuum cleaners only absorb larger particles, and they allow many allergens to escape in the exhaust. This is often why you may experience asthma symptoms after housework: The vacuuming may actually have made matters worse for you by stirring up triggering substances that you then inhaled.

In order to avoid stirring up asthma triggers when you vacuum, ask your doctor whether she thinks investing in a vacuum cleaner that uses a HEPA or ULPA filtration process may work for you.

Working Out Workplace Exposures

Exposures to many types of chemicals and dust in workplace environments can induce different forms of occupational asthma. In many cases, people who have asthma but haven't yet developed obvious symptoms of the disease may experience asthma episodes for the first time as a result of exposure to occupational triggers. Allergic and nonallergic triggers can play a part in occupational asthma, which may account for as many as 15 percent of all new asthma cases each year in the United States.

Targeting workplace triggers

Doctors and other healthcare professionals typically associate occupational asthma with exposure to the following workplace triggers:

✔ **Industrial irritants:** These irritants can include chemicals, fumes, gases, aerosols, paints, smoke, and other substances you primarily find in the workplace. Tobacco smoke in the workplace can cause many asthma symptoms.

Likewise, other irritants in the workplace can include food odors, and even co-workers who use heavily scented perfumes and colognes.

- **Occupational allergens:** Many occupations involve exposure to or contact with substances made of plant materials, food products, and other items that contain allergenic extracts that can trigger allergic reactions, thus inducing occupational asthma in sensitized people. For example, "Baker's asthma" can occur in workers who receive constant respiratory exposure to the allergens contained in flour. (Eating the resulting baked food usually doesn't produce symptoms in these workers, however.) Latex is another common occupational allergen.

- **Physical stimuli:** These stimuli include conditions in your workplace, especially variations in temperature and humidity, such as heat and cold extremes or air that's especially dry or humid.

Diagnosing and treating workplace triggers

Your physician should distinguish between asthma that results from exposure to certain substances in the workplace, school, or other frequented locations (other than your home) and a pre-existing condition aggravated by occupational allergens and irritants. This determination is vital to developing effective methods of avoiding or reducing your exposure to occupational substances that may affect your asthma.

Diagnosing your occupational asthma is important for your long-term health and the effective management of your disease. The sooner you can effectively avoid or reduce your exposure to triggers at work, the better you can control your asthma.

In diagnosing a case of occupational asthma, your doctor may first need to assess the following factors:

- ✓ **The pattern of your symptoms.** Symptoms that improve when you're away from work strongly suggest that your problem is work-related.

- ✓ **Your co-workers.** Do your co-workers suffer from similar symptoms?

- ✓ **The degree of exposure.** Did your first notice-able asthma episode at work occur after a par-ticularly significant exposure, such as a spill of chemicals or other industrial substances?

 Depending on your condition's severity, your doctor may prescribe medications that control your asthma symptoms at work. In most cases, however, for this treatment to be effective, your doctor will probably advise you to find ways of avoiding or at least reducing your exposure to workplace triggers.

Avoiding Drug and Food Triggers

Some people with asthma also suffer from sensitivities — sometimes potentially life-threatening — to certain foods and medications. In the following sections, I explain the most significant sensitivities that can adversely affect your asthma and what you can do to avoid them.

Aspirin sensitivities

Approximately 10 percent of asthma patients experi-ence some level of sensitivity to aspirin, aspirin-containing compounds (such as Alka-Seltzer, Anacin, and Excedrin), and nonsteroidal anti-inflammatory drugs (NSAIDs). If your medical history includes nasal polyps and sinusitis in addition to asthma and aspirin sensitivity, use acetaminophen-based products such as Tylenol rather than aspirin or NSAIDs for the relief of common aches and pains.

A more serious form of aspirin sensitivity is the *aspirin triad.* This condition affects aspirin-intolerant patients who have asthma and chronic nasal polyps as well as a history of sinusitis. If you suffer from the aspirin triad, adverse reactions to aspirin, aspirin-containing compounds, NSAIDs, and prescription NSAIDs, known as COX-2 inhibitors, including celecoxib (Celebrex), can result in severe or potentially life-threatening asthma attacks.

I strongly advise anyone with this level of sensitivity to wear a MedicAlert bracelet or pendant. This device alerts medical personnel not to administer any medication to which you are sensitive if you're unconscious or unable to communicate during a medical emergency.

Beta-blockers

Doctors frequently prescribe oral beta-blocker medications, including Inderal, Lopressor, and Corgard, to treat conditions such as migraine headache, high blood pressure, angina, or hyperthyroidism, and beta-blocker eye drops for eye conditions, such as glaucoma. If you have one of these disorders and you also have asthma, know that taking beta-blockers can worsen your asthma symptoms by blocking the $beta_2$-adrenergic receptor sites in your airways that cause bronchodilation, thus making your asthma less responsive to $beta_2$-adrenergic ($beta_2$-agonist) bronchodilators.

Occasionally, taking beta-blockers can trigger asthma episodes in susceptible individuals who haven't previously experienced any respiratory symptoms.

 Because beta-blockers may trigger asthma symptoms, make sure that any doctor you consult for any of the conditions I mention in this section knows that you have asthma and/or has your complete medical history. If beta-blockers aren't advisable, your doctor may prescribe alternative forms of medication therapy, such as other families of anti-hypertensives or other types of anti-migraine drugs.

Sensitivities to sulfites and other additives

Sulfites are often used as antioxidants to preserve beverages, such as beer and wine, and foods like dried fruit, shrimp, and potatoes. These antioxidants are also often used in salad bars and in guacamole. Exposure to these food additives can trigger severe asthma symptoms — including potentially life-threatening *bronchospasm* (constriction of the airways) — in as many as 10 percent of people who have severe persistent asthma when these individuals inhale sulfite fumes from treated foods. Severe asthmatics who require long-term treatment with oral corticosteroids are more likely to be sulfite-sensitive and may be especially at risk for severe adverse reactions to these additives.

 If you're sensitive to sulfites, avoid consuming beer, wine, and processed foods. Also, carry rescue medication, such as an EpiPen, Twinject, and/or a short-acting inhaled bronchodilator, with you in the event that you unintentionally ingest food or liquids that contain sulfites.

Eating more fresh foods, rather than processed foods, particularly fruits and vegetables, is a good idea anyway, regardless of whether you have asthma.

 Tartrazine (FDC yellow dye No. 5), used in many medications, foods, and vitamin products, has been reported to possibly cause adverse reactions in asthmatics. If you're sensitive to this food additive, check the labels on liquid medications, such as cough syrups and other liquid cold and flu remedies, to see whether they contain tartrazine or sulfites. When in doubt, ask your pharmacist.

Food allergies

Some people with asthma develop hypersensitivities to certain foods. Although certain foods have the potential to cause anaphylaxis, they don't appear to significantly increase the underlying airway inflammation characteristic of asthma in most patients.

 If your infant or young child has food allergies, he or she may have a tendency to develop other allergy-related problems. In this case, your doctor should evaluate your child for possible signs of asthma and other atopic diseases, such as allergic rhinitis and atopic dermatitis.

 If you've experienced an episode of anaphylaxis, ask your doctor whether an emergency epinephrine kit, such as an EpiPen (or EpiPen Jr. for children under 66 pounds) or Twinject, is advisable for you. Wear a MedicAlert bracelet or necklace in case you're unable to speak during a reaction.

Exercise-Induced Asthma

You don't have to sit on life's sidelines just because you have asthma, even though most asthmatics are susceptible, in varying degrees, to symptoms of *exercise-induced asthma* (EIA — also known as *exercise-induced bronchospasm* or EIB).

Typically, EIA symptoms start minutes after you begin vigorous activity, when the airways in your lungs become narrow and constricted. These respiratory symptoms usually reach their peak of severity between five and ten minutes after you stop exercising. In many cases, the symptoms can spontaneously resolve (without the use of a short-acting inhaled bronchodilator) within 30 minutes.

Exercises that involve breathing cold, dry air, such as running outdoors or skiing, are more likely to trigger EIA than activities that involve breathing warmer, humidified air, such as swimming in a heated pool. However, a few studies have cautioned that chlorine and other chemicals used in heated and non-heated pools seem to act as EIA triggers in some asthmatics.

 Although EIA usually relates to outside activities, using home-exercise equipment or simply running up stairs can precipitate an asthma episode in some people. If you have an increased sensitivity for EIA, make sure that your doctor knows so that he can evaluate and treat your condition.

Keeping fit despite EIA

Although EIA symptoms occur frequently in asthmatics when they exert themselves vigorously, for certain individuals, physical activity may be the only trigger that precipitates respiratory symptoms such as coughing, wheezing, and shortness of breath. Occasionally, patients mistakenly attribute their EIA symptoms to just "being out of shape," instead of seeking a proper medical diagnosis.

 If you're experiencing respiratory symptoms connected to exercise and other types of intensive physical activities, make sure that you get a proper diagnosis. Although EIA episodes usually last for only a few minutes, they can still be frightening for many people and, as a result, can unnecessarily limit your physical activities.

Properly diagnosing and treating EIA usually means that you can enjoy an active lifestyle. Doctors can often prescribe medications to prevent or at least substantially reduce your EIA symptoms, thus allowing you to participate in many types of exercise and sports in spite of your asthma.

Receiving appropriate treatment for EIA is also essential for your well-being because so many people in the United States and other developed countries simply don't get enough exercise. According to a recent report by the Centers for Disease Control and Prevention (CDC), adult asthmatics in the U.S. are even less likely on average to meet national recommendations for physical activity than nonasthmatics.

I'm not suggesting you run a marathon tomorrow, but staying in good physical shape can only help in managing your asthma (and any other ailment) successfully. Don't let your susceptibility to EIA keep you from getting the exercise you need; consult with your doctor to find effective ways of managing your condition that also allow you to stay in shape.

 Keeping a record of your activities and noting when you experience asthma symptoms and what steps you normally take to relieve them can assist your doctor in developing the most effective treatment program. Because certain drugs are more effective in preventing and controlling EIA, *when* you take your prescribed medication is often just as important as *what* you take. Work with your doctor to determine the best time to take your prescribed medication in order to ensure that it provides maximum relief.

In many cases, competitive athletes with asthma or EIA use inhaled corticosteroids daily to control their airway inflammation. Many competitive athletes also add a long-acting inhaled beta$_2$-adrenergic bronchodilator daily, such as salmeterol (Serevent, Serevent Diskus) or formoterol (Foradil), and/or a short-acting inhaled beta$_2$-adrenergic bronchodilator, such as albuterol (Proventil, Ventolin), prior to exercise or athletic events.

 To prevent EIA, your doctor may recommend that you inhale your dose of prescribed short-acting beta$_2$-adrenergic bronchodilator 15 to 30 minutes before you begin to exert yourself. The long-acting bronchodilators salmeterol — available in dry-powder inhaler (DPI) formulation as Serevent Diskus or as Serevent MDI in a metered-dose inhaler (MDI) — and formoterol — available only as a DPI as Foradil Aerolizer — may be prescribed for use 30 minutes before exercising. Doctors usually prescribe these medications as part of combination therapy with inhaled corticosteroids. (See Chapter 5 for the differences between DPIs and MDIs.)

Other long-term controller drugs that doctors prescribe to treat EIA symptoms include cromolyn (Intal) and nedocromil (Tilade), which are both inhaled mast cell stabilizers. These products are also usually best taken 15 to 30 minutes before exercising. Recent studies have shown that when taken regularly, montelukast (Singulair), a leukotriene inhibitor, may also be an effective long-term, preventive treatment for EIA.

Athletes and EIA

According to recent studies of respiratory conditions, Olympic-level competitors as a group are most likely to experience EIA episodes. Research indicates that hard breathing by these competitors during sports events and intensive workouts may be an important factor in triggering their respiratory symptoms.

Another reason for athletes being at increased risk for EIA is due to the fact that all people — not just Olympic champions — switch from nose breathing to mouth breathing when they're strenuously exerting themselves. One of your nose's most important functions is to protect your airways from particulate matter in the air. Your nose acts to filter and cleanse the air you inhale, through *cilia* (tiny hairlike projections of certain types of cells that sweep mucus through the nose).

Filtering isn't in your mouth's job description. When you're seriously exerting yourself and gulping in air through your mouth, you're also increasing the chances of inhaling allergens and irritants that can more easily get into the airways of your lungs and potentially trigger more serious reactions.

Because your body needs all the oxygen it can get when you're vigorously working out and/or competing, breathing through your mouth can virtually be a reflex, which is all the more reason to make sure that you're taking medications to prevent or at least reduce the severity of EIA symptoms.

Contrary to popular myth, sports federations such as the National Collegiate Athletic Association (NCAA) or the U.S. Olympic Committee haven't banned the use of inhaled corticosteroids that athletes take on a regular basis to control asthma symptoms. (The steroids that various sports committees ban are actually male hormones that some athletes take by tablet or injection to build muscle mass.) However, some common over-the-counter (OTC) medications, such as pseudoephedrine (Sudafed), are banned due to their stimulant effects. Check with your sports federation before taking any medication, including OTC products.

Many doctors also advise some type of warm-up and cool-down routine (even if you don't have asthma) when engaging in exercise or sports-related activity. Consult with your physician to determine the type of pre- and post-exercise routine that's most beneficial for you.

Other Conditions and Asthma

In addition to the triggers that I discuss previously in this chapter, certain illnesses and syndromes can also induce your asthma symptoms or make them worse. Managing these precipitating factors is vital to effectively controlling your asthma.

Rhinitis and sinusitis

Poorly managing allergic and nonallergic forms of rhinitis can lead to *sinusitis*. This infection of the sinuses can also aggravate your asthma symptoms, especially if it isn't responsive to repeated courses of antibiotic treatment. If so, sinus surgery may be necessary to treat sinusitis and reestablish control over asthma symptoms. Studies show that asthma patients who effectively manage their rhinitis and/or sinusitis can significantly improve their asthma symptoms.

Because your respiratory tract is essentially a continuum — or as I like to say, the united airway — treating your nose and sinuses can actually help treat the underlying inflammation that characterizes asthma. In fact, when dealing with serious respiratory diseases such as asthma, doctors increasingly consider it vital to treat the whole patient — not just the patient's lungs.

Gastroesophageal reflux disease

 The digestive disorder *gastroesophageal reflux disease* (GERD) occurs when the valve that separates the esophagus from the stomach doesn't function properly. As a result, stomach acid and undigested food can wash up into the esophagus (and occasionally, through inhalation, into the respiratory tract) from the stomach in individuals who suffer from GERD. See a cross section of the organs involved in GERD in Figure 3-1.

Patients who suffer from GERD often burp during and after meals, complain of an acid taste in their mouth, and feel a burning sensation in their throat or chest, symptoms that they typically describe as heartburn or indigestion.

GERD is a trigger of asthma symptoms in a large number of asthmatics, and is, in particular, a major trigger of adult-onset asthma (see Chapter 1) in patients whose asthma symptoms (coughing, wheezing, shortness of breath) aren't usually associated with allergic triggers. If you're asthmatic, the flow of acidic digestive contents into your respiratory airways can make your underlying airway inflammation worse. GERD, with or without inhalation of stomach contents, has also been associated with increased bronchospasm and chronic cough due to irritation of the esophagus. Conversely, when asthma is active, it can also aggravate GERD, and some of the drugs used to treat asthma, such as long-acting $beta_2$-adrenergic bronchodilators and oral theophylline, can also worsen GERD symptoms.

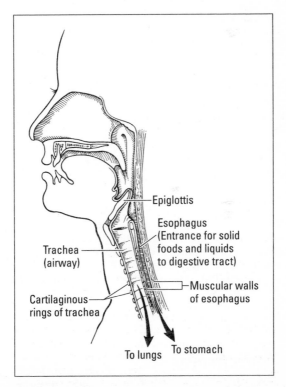

Epiglottis

Esophagus
(Entrance for solid
foods and liquids
to digestive tract)

Trachea
(airway)

Muscular walls
of esophagus

Cartilaginous
rings of trachea

To lungs   To stomach

Figure 3-1: GERD occurs when stomach contents spill over into the trachea.

If you have frequent heartburn and poorly controlled asthma, particularly with episodes that
occur at night and disturb your sleep, your
doctor should investigate the possibility that
GERD contributes to your asthma symptoms.

To help alleviate the effects of GERD, your doctor may
advise the following:

- ✔ Avoid eating or drinking within three hours of
  going to bed.

- ✔ Avoid heavy meals and minimize dietary fat.
  Also, try to eat several small meals over the
  course of the day rather than fewer, larger meals.

- ✔ Eliminate or cut down on the consumption of
  chocolate, peppermint, alcoholic beverages,
  coffee, tea, and colas and carbonated beverages.

- ✔ Avoid or reduce smoking and the use of any
  tobacco products.

- ✔ Try elevating the head of your bed, by using 6-
  to 8-inch blocks, so that your stomach contents
  are less likely to rise to the point that you can
  inhale them while sleeping. Adding pillows
  under your head can also be of some benefit.

- ✔ To control the digestive problems that result
  from your GERD symptoms, use appropriate
  over-the-counter (OTC) products, including
  Zantac, Tagamet, Axid, Prilosec OTC, and
  Pepcid AC. Your physician may also prescribe
  other medications, such as Nexium, Protonix,
  Aciphex, and Prevacid, which decrease *gastric*
  (stomach) acid secretion.

Viral infections

Viral respiratory infections, such as the common cold
or flu, can aggravate airway inflammation and trigger

asthma symptoms. Asthmatic children under age 10 are particularly prone to asthma symptoms precipitated by *rhinovirus infections* (upper respiratory infections, usually referred to as the common cold).

Rhinovirus infections cause bronchial hyperreactivity and promote allergic inflammation, leading to increased asthma symptoms. For infants and toddlers, viral infections of all types are the most frequent cause of severe asthma episodes because infants and younger children have smaller airways that are often more susceptible to bronchial obstruction. These infections are also the most frequent cause of episodes in adults, especially those with nonallergic (intrinsic) asthma.

 Inform your doctor whenever you experience flu or cold symptoms. As comforting as you may find chicken soup when you're sneezy, you may require early and aggressive medication therapy to keep the virus from adversely affecting your asthma.

Consider the following measures when dealing with viral infections:

✔ If you have persistent asthma, ask your doctor about receiving an annual flu vaccine to reduce the risk of suffering from an influenza respiratory infection that could aggravate your asthma symptoms.

✔ New prescription antiviral medications, such as zanamivir by inhalation (Relenza) and oseltamivir phosphate by oral tablet (Tamiflu), can stop the flu dead in its tracks and get you back on your feet sooner if you take them within the first two days of developing flu symptoms. Common flu symptoms include high fever, muscle aches, fatigue, and increased respiratory symptoms. Using these antiviral products can reduce the respiratory complications that accompany influenza infections, making these medications especially beneficial if you have asthma. However, these medications are only for influenza and aren't effective against the common cold.

✔ If your young child or infant experiences repeated viral infections that cause coughing and wheezing episodes, and your family medical history includes *atopy* (the genetic susceptibility for the immune system to produce antibodies to common allergens, which leads to allergy symptoms), make sure your doctor evaluates your child for the possibility of asthma.

Chapter 4

Avoiding Allergens That Cause Respiratory Symptoms

. . . .

In This Chapter

▶ Understanding pollen and mold

▶ Minding mites and other dusty denizens

▶ Eliminating, controlling, and avoiding allergens and irritants in your home

. . . .

*U*nder normal circumstances, breathing is a reflex you don't even think about — as long as nothing in the air interferes with the process. However, unless you live in a bubble, every time you breathe in, you inhale more than oxygen into your nose and lungs.

In fact, the air that most people breathe is full of many types of airborne particles that are too small for the naked eye to see. In addition to pollutants and other airborne materials, these particles include allergenic substances, known as *aeroallergens,* that can trigger allergic reactions and significantly affect the well-being of people with asthma or allergies. The inhaled aeroallergens that trigger allergic reactions are known as *inhalant allergens.*

In this chapter, I give you the lowdown on common inhalant allergens and explain the dangers of each in detail. I also discuss ways you can avoid or at least limit your exposure to these allergens.

Pollens

Pollens can trigger allergic rhinitis (also known as hay fever) and asthma symptoms. Plants that depend on wind rather than insects for pollination produce pollens. These plants release their wind-borne pollens in huge quantities to reproduce.

Pollen particulars

A variety of means, including insects, animals, and the wind, provide transportation for pollen granules. Wind-borne pollens that trigger allergic rhinitis symptoms come from three classifications of plants:

✔ **Grasses:** The grasses that cause most grass-induced allergic rhinitis are widespread throughout North America and were imported from Europe to feed animals and create lawns. By contrast, the many native grasses of North America produce little pollen. I provide more details on these grasses in the "Allergens in the grass" section, later in this chapter.

✔ **Weeds:** The most important weeds that trigger symptoms of allergic rhinitis are those of the tribe *Ambrosieae,* known as *ragweeds.*

✔ **Trees:** Most trees that release symptom-causing pollens are *angiosperms* (which means "flowering seeds," yet these trees don't actually flower), such as willows, poplars, beeches, and oaks. Similarly, pollens from a few *gymnosperms*

(naked seeds), such as pines, spruces, firs,
junipers, cypresses, hemlocks, and cedars, also
can trigger symptoms.

Although these plant groups account for most cases
of pollen-induced allergic rhinitis, only a small percentage of the members of each group has been shown to
produce allergenic pollen.

Most wind-pollinating plants in the United States and
Canada release pollens at specific times during the
year that can be classified into five pollen seasons.
Whenever your respiratory symptoms begin or worsen
during one of these seasons, the predominance of
particular pollens during that particular time of year
may be the cause of allergic reactions that complicate
your asthma. Here's the type of pollen (or molds) that
may affect you in each of the five pollen seasons:

- ✔ When your symptoms get worse during spring,
  the probable cause is tree pollen.

- ✔ In late spring and early summer, grass pollen is
  the likely culprit.

- ✔ From late summer to autumn, weed pollen,
  especially from ragweed, may cause problems.

- ✔ Especially during the summer and fall but also
  throughout the year — except during snow
  cover — mold spores, particularly those of
  airborne molds, may trigger allergies.

- ✔ In winter, wind-borne pollens rarely are a factor
  in most parts of the United States and Canada.
  However, in the warmer southern regions of the
  United States that don't experience prolonged
  periods of freezing temperatures (such as southern California), pollinating plants and molds still
  release allergy-triggering pollen and mold spores
  whenever snow cover is absent.

When your allergic rhinitis symptoms follow a seasonal pattern, such as those I just listed, consult your doctor to find out whether specific pollens are the problem. You may also want to ask for information on the major aeroallergens for the area 50 to 100 miles around where you live and work.

A list of local allergenic plants can serve as a good starting point for figuring out what plants may be affecting your allergies. However, knowing about non-native plants in your environment also is useful. Non-native plants in your environment often include trees and grasses — some of which may also produce allergenic pollen — that may have been planted around your community for decorative purposes.

Counting your pollens

Many newspapers and television and radio news programs regularly report *pollen counts.* The pollen count is the measurement of the total number of granules of a kind of particular pollen per cubic meter of air per day. Pollen counters rate the resulting numbers according to five categories, ranging from absent to very high.

Bear in mind that the severity of symptoms triggered by pollens depends not only on the actual pollen count but also on the particular pollen being measured. In addition, the proximity of the collection station to the particular pollen being reported usually affects the actual count; moreover, each region of the world has its own predominant allergy-producing pollens. Table 4-1 provides the generally accepted guidelines for interpreting pollen counts for ragweed, which is the most closely-followed type of pollen count in many parts of the United States and Canada.

Table 4-1	Ragweed Pollen Count Guidelines	
Category	*Pollen Grains Per Cubic Meter Per Day**	*Degree of Symptoms*
Absent	0	No symptoms.
Low	0–10	Symptoms may only affect people with extreme sensitivities to these pollens.
Moderate	10–50	Many people who are sensitive to these pollens experience symptoms at this rating.
High	50–500	Most people with any sensitivity to these pollens experience symptoms.
Very High	More than 500	Almost anyone with any sensitivity at all to these pollens experiences symptoms. If you're extremely sensitive to ragweed pollen, your symptoms can be severe at this level.

*These figures are averages.

When you read a pollen count, keep in mind these other factors:

✔ Today's pollen count was collected yesterday and reflects what was in the air 24 hours ago.

✔ Rain can clear pollen out of the air temporarily. However, short thunderstorms — characteristic of late spring and summer in parts of North America — can actually spread pollen granules farther.

✔ Hot weather increases pollination, whereas cooler temperatures reduce the amount of pollen that plants produce.

✔ Pollen grains typically are at their highest concentrations from mid-morning to early afternoon.

✔ Because they're wind-borne, many pollen granules travel great distances, so the plants in your yard may not be triggering your allergies.

Not all pollens are equal. Studies show that a little pollen from grasses such as Bermuda and bluegrass or trees such as oak and elm can go a long way in triggering allergies. On the other hand, allergic rhinitis symptoms usually are triggered only by much higher and direct exposures to pine and eucalyptus pollen. These pollens are large and heavy and don't disperse widely in the wind. So knowing the types of pollens blowing in the wind, and how much of those pollens are actually in the wind, is important.

Consider these tips to help you minimize problems during those high pollen–count days:

✔ Whenever your community reports high counts for pollens to which you're allergic, you can take steps to avoid or reduce your exposure to those pollens. For details on how, see the "Pollen-proofing" section, later in this chapter.

✔ If complete or significant avoidance isn't practical or possible, you can use pollen counts to help you determine (based on your doctor's advice) when to take medication to prevent the onset of symptoms or at least keep them from interfering dramatically with your life.

✔ The most important pollen levels for you to consider are the ones that trigger your allergies.

Many people react differently to different levels of airborne pollen, and pollens vary between regions. However, you need to be concerned when pollen counts reach the moderate range, because that's generally when many people with allergies start to experience symptoms.

Contact the National Allergy Bureau (NAB) of the American Academy of Allergy, Asthma, and Immunology (AAAAI) for info about the pollens and molds in your area. Check out the NAB Web site at www.aaaai.org/nab or call 414-272-6071.

Allergens in the grass

Grass pollens are the most common cause of allergies in the world. Although only a small percentage of the more than 1,000 species of grasses in North America actually produce pollen that triggers asthma symptoms and allergic reactions, these particular species are widespread throughout the continent and release huge amounts of pollen granules into the air. Most of these grasses are non-native plants that were imported to grow feed for farm animals and for planting lawns.

Wind-pollinated grasses release vast amounts of pollen granules during the late spring pollen season. The most significant allergy-symptom provoking grasses are Bermuda grass, bluegrass, orchard grass, ryegrass, timothy, and fescue. Of those grasses, Bermuda grass may be the most significant allergy trigger. Bermuda grass releases pollen almost year-round and abounds throughout the southern United States, where it's cultivated for ornamental purposes and as animal feed. Other grasses, such as rye, timothy, blue, and orchard, share allergens in common, so an allergy to pollen from one of these grasses may also indicate sensitivity to allergens from one or more of these other grasses.

Wheezy weeds

When I refer to *weeds,* I mean the small, wild, annual plants of no agricultural value or decorative interest. The wind-pollinated weeds that release allergenic pollen don't produce very attractive or conspicuous flowers. The most significant of these wind-pollinated weeds, in terms of allergic triggers, include ragweed, mugwort, Russian thistle, pigweed, sagebrush, and English plantain.

 Ragweed is a significant trigger of asthma symptoms and is the most common cause of allergic rhinitis reactions in North America. Many people who are sensitive to ragweed may also experience cross-reactivity to cocklebur.

In the United States, from the mid-Atlantic to northern parts of the Midwest, where ragweed is most highly concentrated, pollination usually begins around August 15 and generally lasts through October (and/ or until a first frost), depending on climate conditions. Ragweeds are early risers, with most plants releasing pollen between 6 and 11 a.m. Hot and humid weather usually leads to an increased release of pollen.

Although ragweed pollen is most prevalent east of the Mississippi River, you can find related weed pollens, such as those produced by marsh elder and cocklebur, throughout most parts of North America.

Can't sneeze the forest for the trees

Of the 700 species of trees that are native to North America, only 65 produce pollen that triggers allergic rhinitis. The pollination season for most of these species usually runs from the end of winter or the beginning of spring until early summer.

Pollens from these types of trees have much shorter ranges than the pollens that wind-pollinating grasses and weeds release. As a result, in most cities and towns, weed and grass pollens are far more likely to affect you than tree pollens. However, in the southeastern United States, the spring tree season is a major problem, with high peaks of pollination over a prolonged period of time.

Trees that produce the most allergenic pollen in North America include elms; willows and poplars; birches; beeches, oaks, and chestnuts; maples and box elders; hickories; mountain cedars; and ashes and olives.

Molds

Talk about moldies and oldies: Molds are some of the oldest and most common organisms on the planet, and they're widespread in most homes. Think of molds as microscopic fungi or mushrooms. You've probably encountered various forms of mold at home, from splotches on your shower door to the greenish growth on that tomato you forgot way in the back of your fridge last year (hope your mom doesn't find out).

Throughout the United States and Canada, mold spores are some of the most common inhalant allergens, outdoors and indoors, and can be significant triggers of asthma, allergic rhinitis, and other respiratory ailments.

Mold counts usually are much higher than pollen counts and usually rise to peak levels during summer months. Outdoor mold spores are present almost year-round unless prolonged snow cover occurs. This mold-spore propensity is in contrast to pollens, which are released by plants, usually only during distinct seasons. However, at any time, mold counts can suddenly and dramatically rise within a short period and then drop down to previous levels just as abruptly. Because molds also thrive indoors, you may be exposed to mold spores continuously during the year.

Outdoor molds grow on field crops such as corn, wheat, soybeans, and on decaying organic matter such as compost, hay, piles of leaves, and grass cuttings, and types of foods, including tomatoes, sweet corn, melons, bananas, and mushrooms.

Spreading spores

Only a few forms of molds produce allergens that trigger asthma and allergic rhinitis symptoms. Airborne mold spores occur almost everywhere on the planet except at the North and South poles. So unless you're a polar bear or a penguin, odds are that you receive some degree of exposure to mold particles, regardless of where you are. These molds include

- ✔ **Cladosporium:** These species produce some of the most abundant wind-borne spores in the world and flourish almost everywhere, except in the coldest regions.

- ✔ **Alternaria:** These outdoor molds are among the most prominent causes of allergy symptoms in sensitized people.

- ✔ **Aspergillus:** A medically important indoor mold, found in agricultural areas, crawl spaces of homes, and outdoor air throughout North America. A variety of allergic respiratory diseases associated with exposure to aspergillus are recognized, including allergic asthma (see Chapter 1), hypersensitivity pneumonitis *(farmer's lung)*, and a serious respiratory disease known as allergic bronchopulmonary aspergillosis (ABPA).

Moldy matters

Here are factors that can help you determine whether mold spores are triggering your respiratory symptoms:

- ✔ You experience asthma symptoms most of the year, rather than during specific seasons.
- ✔ Your symptoms worsen during summer months, even when pollen allergens aren't present to any significant degree.
- ✔ Your asthma worsens near croplands, especially around grains and overgrown fields, or during or immediately following gardening.

House Dust

House dust may be the most prevalent of all triggers of respiratory symptoms in your life. Recent studies show that the major inhalant allergens found in house dust can be the most important risk factors in triggering asthma attacks.

Let me reassure you: Dust isn't dirt, and it isn't an indication of poor housekeeping. Household dust is inescapable because it's a normal breakdown product of fibers and other materials found throughout your indoor environment. Common components of house dust include

- ✔ Dust mite allergens
- ✔ Animal dander
- ✔ Insect fragments
- ✔ Fibers such as acrylic, rayon, nylon, and cotton
- ✔ Wood and paper particles
- ✔ Hair and skin flakes

✔ Tobacco ash

✔ Particles of salt, sugar, other spices, and minerals

✔ Plant pollen and fungal spores

Dust mites

The most potent allergen in house dust comes from the house dust mite. These tiny, eight-legged microscopic spider relatives live in house dust where they feed on dead skin flakes that warm-blooded creatures such as humans constantly shed at rates of up to 1.5 grams per day — that's a lot of dust mite chow.

The fecal matter (or waste, to put it more delicately) that they produce, at the average rate of 20 particles per day, is the most prevalent form of house dust allergens and often causes respiratory problems in humans.

Because dust mites usually are as snug as bugs in a rug, people rarely come into direct contact with the live creatures themselves — just with their waste or decomposing bodies, which also can be a significant source of house dust allergens. Dust mites thrive in dark, warm, and humid environments such as mattresses, pillows, box springs, rugs, towels, upholstered furniture, drapes, and stuffed toys.

Mattresses and box springs usually provide the greatest concentration of human skin flakes for these creatures, which is why the average bed contains 2 million dust mites. As a result, your asthma symptoms may worsen in bed or while napping on your upholstered couch, because you inhale significant amounts of dust mite allergens while sleeping. That's why many of the steps that I recommend for your home in the section about "Avoidance and Allergy-Proofing," later in this chapter, focus on your bedroom.

What else is in my house dust?

Although you may not have pets of your own, whenever you're in contact with other pet owners, dander from their animals can get on your hands or clothes, which you then introduce into your home. In addition, the urine from household pests, such as mice and rats, can be significant triggers of asthma symptoms. Furthermore, recent studies increasingly show that allergens in cockroach debris and waste can contribute to asthma attacks, especially in children.

Is dust my problem?

The following is a list of symptoms that you can use to determine whether inhalant allergens in house dust trigger your respiratory symptoms:

- ✔ You experience symptoms as a result of dusting, making beds, or changing blankets and bed linens.

- ✔ Your symptoms seem to occur year-round rather than seasonally.

- ✔ Your symptoms are worse when you're indoors.

- ✔ Your symptoms are worse when you awaken in bed in the morning.

Avoidance and Allergy-Proofing

In the first part of this chapter, I tell you about the most important and prevalent triggers of respiratory symptoms that affect most asthma patients. In the rest of the chapter, I discuss steps you can take to avoid — or at least significantly decrease your exposure to — those triggers. These methods usually help you improve your life with asthma.

Why avoidance matters

You've probably heard the joke about the patient who complains, "Doc, it hurts when I do this," to which the doctor replies, "Then stop doing that." (For more great doctor jokes, come to one of my book signings.) Silly as that joke seems, the doctor's advice exemplifies the basic concept of avoidance. Depending on your sensitivity, avoid the substances or levels of exposure to the substances that trigger (that's why such substances are called *triggers*) an allergic reaction.

Avoidance seems simple enough. In real life, however, the trick is figuring out — short of living in a bubble — the practical and effective steps you can take to minimize your contact with triggers.

Environmental control measures are vital components of any allergist's treatment plan. Every practicing allergist focuses on helping you create and implement an effective avoidance strategy for you, your spouse, your child, or other people with asthma who live with you. The plan that you and your allergist develop will likely include these general steps:

1. **Identifying asthma and allergy triggers in your environment, especially indoor allergens and irritants.**

2. **Recognizing situations in which you may come into contact with those allergy triggers.**

3. **Discovering how to avoid allergens or minimizing contact with them.**

4. **Allergy-proofing your home.**

 In case you're also allergic to jargon, the following list explains common technical terms that allergists use when discussing avoidance and allergy-proofing:

✔ **Allergen load:** Your total level of exposure, at any given time, to any combination of allergens that trigger your allergies.

✔ **Allergic threshold:** Your level of sensitivity to an allergen. A low allergic threshold means that your sensitivity to an allergen is high — even a small exposure to the substance can trigger your symptoms. A high allergic threshold means that your body requires a higher concentration of allergens to trigger symptoms. Your threshold level, however, can decrease when you're exposed too often to large quantities of an allergen or to a combination of allergens.

✔ **Allergy trigger:** A normally harmless substance, such as pollen, dust, animal dander, insect stings, and certain foods and drugs, that can provoke an abnormal response by your immune system whenever you're sensitized to that substance. Doctors usually refer to these substances as *allergens.*

✔ **Cross-reactivity:** Your immune system is an expert at recognizing related allergens in seemingly unrelated sources. Therefore, if you're exposed to related allergens within a short time, your allergen load can exceed your allergic threshold, thereby triggering allergic reactions and asthma symptoms.

✔ **Desensitization:** In the context of avoidance and allergy-proofing, *desensitizing* describes the active process of removing, shielding, or reducing the sources of allergens in your environment. Your allergist may advise you to desensitize your home, focusing on the bedroom of any person with asthma. *Desensitization* also refers to a form of treatment in which an allergist injects small amounts of an allergen extract under your skin so that your body can discover how not to react to the substance.

✔ **HEPA:** HEPA stands for high efficiency particulate arrester — an air filtration process developed for hospital operating rooms and other locations that require a sterilized environment. HEPA filters absorb and contain 99.97 percent of all particles larger than 0.3 microns ($\frac{1}{300}$ the width of a human hair). When the unit truly operates at that level, only 3 of 10,000 particles manage to sneak back into the room. Vacuum cleaners and air purifiers with ULPA (see definition later in this list) and HEPA filters are vital tools for desensitizing and allergy-proofing your indoor environment.

✔ **HVAC:** Heating, ventilation, and air-conditioning systems — your home's lungs. The quality of air that you breathe indoors is largely dependent on the condition of these systems and the air that flows into and out of your environment through them.

✔ **ULPA:** Ultra low penetration air is even more thorough than the HEPA process. This filtration system is designed to absorb and contain 99.99 percent of all particles larger than 0.12 microns.

Knowing your limits

Avoidance measures rarely require the complete elimination of all asthma and allergy triggers and irritants in your environment. In many cases, you may need only to limit your exposure to certain triggers to prevent or alleviate your respiratory symptoms.

Think of your allergic threshold as a cup and the allergy triggers in your environment as liquid pouring into the cup. Overflowing your small cup (low allergic threshold) may require only a small amount of liquid (allergens), thereby triggering an allergic reaction. A larger cup — a higher threshold — can accommodate more liquid without overflowing (without triggering an allergic reaction). Knowing your limit is the key to mastering your threshold.

Another important concept to bear in mind when considering avoidance is imagining a scale balancing your allergic threshold on one side with allergen load on the other. You won't set off your allergies unless your level of exposure to allergen triggers overloads your allergic threshold. Keep in mind, however, that your scales can tip not only from excessive exposure to a single allergen but also from exposure to small amounts of a variety of allergens.

Crossing the line

Cross-reactivity also is an important factor in causing allergic reactions and asthma symptoms. It can contribute toward overloading your allergic threshold. For example, when you have sensitivity to ragweed, you may also be sensitive to allergens in melons — honeydew, cantaloupe, and watermelon.

This phenomenon occurs because, in some individuals, an allergenic cross-reactivity that exists between certain food proteins and nonfood protein sources can look similar to their immune systems. As a result, in addition to ragweed allergy symptoms during ragweed season, you may also experience itching and swelling of your mouth and lips when eating melons, even though these fruits may not present a problem for you during the rest of the year. Some people also experience cross-reactivity reactions between latex and — of all things — bananas, avocados, papaya, kiwi, and chestnuts.

The Great Indoors

One downside of modern structures is that indoor environments — at home, work, school, and even in cars and other enclosed means of transportation — can often contain far more significant sources of asthma and allergy triggers than outdoor environments. Irritants and allergens can concentrate in most enclosures, and because people spend so much time indoors, that's where they often experience the most significant exposure to allergy triggers.

If you have asthma and/or allergic rhinitis, you may focus your attention solely on pollen counts, air pollution, and other elements of the outdoor environment as the prime sources for allergens and irritants that trigger your symptoms and reactions. You may also assume that indoor air is cleaner and safer than the air that you breathe outside. However, according to Environmental Protection Agency studies, indoor air can actually contain as much as 70 times the pollution of outdoor air.

According to the American Lung Association, most people spend 90 percent of their time indoors, spending 60 percent of that time at home. Therefore, indoor air pollution is a serious concern for everyone, particularly because studies show that it can cause or aggravate asthma and allergies.

Allergy-Proofing at Home

Although I certainly advise you to avoid or limit exposure to allergens and irritants outside, at work, at school, or in other indoor locations, avoidance therapy actually can have the most beneficial impact in your home. Even when you're exposed to allergy triggers outside your home, reducing your exposure to those allergens and irritants at home may prevent your allergen threshold from overloading.

On average, most people spend a third of their lives in the bedroom — much of that time in bed. As a result, the bedroom is the most important single area of your home. After allergy-proofing your bedroom, try using it as much as possible to ensure that you give your allergies a rest.

In and around your home, the most common and important sources of allergens that you need to focus on when allergy-proofing are

✔ Dust and dust mites

✔ Pets

✔ Mold

✔ Pollen

Controlling irritants at home also is vital to successful avoidance therapy. Although these substances don't trigger allergic responses by your body's immune system (as is the case with allergens), they often worsen existing asthma or allergy conditions.

 Tobacco smoke is the most significant irritant found in the home that aggravates allergy and asthma reactions. Other important irritants include

✔ Aerosols, paints, and smoke from wood-burning stoves

✔ Glue

✔ Household cleaners

✔ Perfumes and scents

✔ Scented soaps

The basics of allergy-proofing are explained in detail in the following sections.

Controlling the dust in your house

Studies show that the average six-room home in the United States collects 40 pounds of dust each year. House dust is one of the most prevalent asthma and allergy triggers in any home, and unfortunately, it's everywhere. Think of house dust as one of life's inevitabilities — along with death and taxes.

Ridding your house of dust mites

Allergy-proofing your bedroom and home likely involves dealing with dust mites more than with any other allergy trigger, because these microscopic creatures produce the single largest component of house dust that triggers respiratory symptoms in asthma patients. Although you've probably never seen them, dust mites are a fact of life — they're bound to follow almost anyplace you settle.

Controlling dust in the bedroom

Few of us ever go to bed alone. Dust mites thrive in dark and humid environments such as mattresses, pillows, and box springs. In fact, the average bed contains 2 million dust mites, which means that you may breathe in significant amounts of dust mite allergens while you sleep. Dust mites also survive well in blankets, carpets, towels, upholstered furniture, drapery, and children's stuffed toys. Although eradication of these natural inhabitants of your home is virtually impossible — the females lay 20 to 50 eggs every three weeks — you can take practical and effective steps to minimize exposure to dust mite allergens.

In my experience, taking the following measures often results in a significant decrease in respiratory symptoms and medication requirements for patients with asthma and allergies:

✔ **Beds:** Encase all pillows, mattresses, and box springs in special allergen-impermeable casings, and mount all beds on bed frames. Wash all bed linens in hot water (at least 130 degrees) every two weeks. Use pillows, blankets, quilts, and bedspreads made of synthetic materials. Avoid down-filled (feather) comforters and pillows.

✔ **Temperature and climate control:** Don't locate your bedroom in a warm (more than 72 degrees), humid area. Likewise, use air conditioners or dehumidifiers to keep the humidity in your home below 50 percent. You may want to use a humidity gauge to monitor humidity levels.

✔ **Carpets and drapes:** Bare surfaces such as hardwood, linoleum, or tile floors are inhospitable to dust mites and are also much easier to clean, thereby minimizing dust buildup. If you can't remove your carpeting and rugs, treat them with products that deactivate dust mite allergens. I also recommend washable curtains or window shades rather than heavy draperies or blinds.

✔ **Housekeeping:** Vacuum thoroughly, at least once a week, with a HEPA or ULPA vacuum cleaner (see the "Why avoidance matters" section, earlier in this chapter). Wear a dust mask when cleaning or engaging in any activity that stirs up dust, and consider cleaning your furniture with a tannic acid solution.

✔ **Ventilation:** Use HEPA air cleaners to keep the indoor air throughout your home as pure as possible. (See the "Why avoidance matters" section, earlier in this chapter.) Cover any heating vents with special vent filters to clean the air before it enters your rooms.

✔ **Decorations and furnishings:** Use furniture made of wood, vinyl, plastic, and leather throughout your home rather than furniture made of upholstery. Likewise, make your bedroom as uncluttered and wipeable as possible. Avoid shelves, pennants, posters, photos, heavy cushions, and other dust collectors. Limit the clothes, books, and other personal objects in your bedroom to the essentials, and make sure that you shut closets or drawers when not in use.

If your child has allergies or asthma, don't turn his or her bedroom into a stuffed animal zoo. Try limiting those toys to a few machine-washable ones. Keep your child's stuffed animals and toys in the closet or in a closed chest, container, or drawer when not in use.

Regulating pet dander

Pets are cherished members of many households. However, *dander* (skin flakes) from these animals is a significant source of allergy triggers for many people. All warm-blooded household pets, regardless of hair length, produce proteins in their dander and saliva that can trigger allergies. Dead skin cells in their dander can even serve as a food supply for dust mites. Cat dander residue can linger at significant exposure levels in carpets for up to 20 weeks and in mattresses for years, even after you remove the animal.

I usually advise people with asthma or allergies not to introduce new pets into their homes. If you already have a pet, I realize that removing this member of the family can be an emotional issue for you and other members, even though Fluffy or Fido's dander may be triggering your respiratory symptoms or those of your children.

If finding a new home for your pet isn't likely, I advise the following measures:

✔ Keep your pet outdoors whenever possible. If keeping your pet outdoors isn't possible, try to keep the pet out of the patient's bedroom. Consider running a HEPA filter 24 hours a day in the bedroom and keeping the door closed.

✔ Make sure that anyone who touches your pet washes his or her hands before contacting the patient or entering the patient's bedroom.

✔ Wash your pet with water once a week. Doing so may remove surface allergens and possibly reduce the amount of dander that can stick to other household members' clothes and bodies (thereby reaching the patient's bedroom).

Controlling mold in your abode

Molds release fungal spores into the air. These spores settle on organic matter and grow into new mold clusters. When inhaled by sensitized individuals, these airborne spores can trigger allergic symptoms. Airborne mold spores are more numerous than pollen grains, and unlike pollen, they don't have a limited season. In parts of the United States and Canada, mold spores may be present until the first snow cover.

Outdoor mold spores can enter your home through the air, by blowing in open windows and doors, and through vents. Indoor molds can grow year-round, and they thrive in dark, humid areas of the home, such as basements and bathrooms. Molds also grow under carpets and in pillows, mattresses, air conditioners, garbage containers, and refrigerators. The older your home, the larger the amount of mold that grows there.

Limiting your exposure to mold spores is a key part of allergy-proofing your home. Take these steps to control molds in and around your home:

✔ Avoid damp areas of your home, such as an unfinished basement or a room with a water leak. Or use a dehumidifier to lower humidity in those areas to 35 percent to 40 percent.

✔ Make sure your clothes dryer vents to the outside.

✔ Ventilate your bathroom well, especially after showers or bathing. Use mold-killing and mold-preventing solutions behind the toilet, around the sink, shower, bathtub, washing machine, and refrigerator, and in other areas of your home where water or moisture collects.

✔ Clean any visible mold from the walls, floors, and ceiling by using a nonchlorine bleach.

✔ Take out the trash and clean your garbage container regularly to prevent mold growth.

✔ Dry out damp footwear and clothing in which mold can breed. Don't hang clothes outside, where mold spores can land on them.

✔ Limit the number of indoor plants or remove them altogether, because mold may grow in potting soil. Dried flowers may also contain mold, so avoid them, too.

 Avoid exposure to outdoor molds around your home. These molds proliferate in fallen leaves, compost, cut grass, fertilizer, hay, and barns. Whenever you work in your yard, wear a well-fitting breathing mask. Cut back any heavy vegetation around your home to let the structure breathe and to prevent dampness and mold growth.

Pollen-proofing

Many people associate allergic rhinitis primarily with outdoor exposure to pollen. You may also experience significant levels of pollen at home, and these exposures also can trigger allergic rhinitis symptoms.

Most pollens are wind-borne; they often blow indoors (typically through open windows and doors) and trigger allergic symptoms, such as allergic rhinitis, within your home and not just outdoors. Wind-pollinated trees, grasses, and weeds produce pollen during various times of the year. (See "Counting your pollens," earlier in this chapter, for details.)

 Take these steps, especially during periods of high pollination, to avoid excessive exposure to pollen:

✔ Avoid intense outdoor activities, such as exercise or strenuous work, during the early morning and late afternoon hours when pollen counts are highest. Whenever you need to work outside, wear a pollen and dust mask.

✔ Close windows and run a HEPA or ULPA air purifier.

✔ Clean and replace your air conditioner filters regularly.

✔ Wash your hair before going to bed to avoid getting pollen on your pillow.

✔ Use a clothes dryer instead of hanging the wash outside where it acts as a filter trap for pollen. You may like the idea of fresh, air-dried laundry, but your target organs won't enjoy the allergic reactions that all the fresh pollen triggers — especially when you hang sheets and pillowcases out on the line.

Chapter 5

Controlling Asthma with Medications

- -

In This Chapter
▶ Adhering to your asthma medication program
▶ Distinguishing between preventive and rescue drugs
▶ Using and maintaining inhalers and nebulizers

- -

*T*reatment with medications, which doctors refer to as *pharmacotherapy,* is a crucial component of your asthma management plan (see Chapter 1). Adhering to your doctor's instructions for taking prescribed medications is vital in effectively treating your condition.

Physicians who care for people with asthma are aware that patients prefer not to take medications on a regular basis. However, asthma is more than the coughing, wheezing, or other symptoms that you may occasionally experience. If you have persistent asthma — like the majority of asthmatics in the United States — some degree of airway inflammation and *hyperreactivity* (increased sensitivity) is always present, even when you aren't noticing any obvious respiratory symptoms and therefore feel fine. Controlling that inflammation is the key to keeping your condition from getting out of hand.

For the vast majority of asthma patients, treatment with at least some form of controller (long-term) and/ or rescue (short-term) medication is almost always an essential component of reducing the severity and frequency of your symptoms, and in some cases even eliminating them and improving your overall quality of life.

Taking Your Medicine

Asthma is a chronic condition requiring chronic treatment. Therefore, treat your asthma the way people with heart disease or diabetes treat their ailments: by taking medications preventively, on a regular basis. Most asthmatics get into trouble with their disease from too little rather than too much treatment. As I explain in Chapter 1, patients who take their medications as directed can prevent the majority of emergency room visits and hospitalizations that asthma causes.

Your physician's goal is to determine the most appropriate medications to help you control your symptoms and achieve your best possible lung function without adverse side effects. Therefore, routinely take the drugs that your doctor prescribes, because they're essential to managing your condition and because they can help significantly improve your quality of life. Without using the medications that your doctor prescribes, you're likely to have a much more difficult time controlling your asthma.

Asthma's changing dynamics

Because asthma is a chronic disease, the vast majority of asthmatics need to take appropriate long-acting, preventive ("controller") medications throughout their lifetime in order to control the underlying airway inflammation that characterizes this disease.

However, asthma is also a dynamic condition. As a result, the combination — and dosages — of medications that your doctor prescribes for you may vary over time. For this reason, consistently consulting your physician about your medication regimen is vital — regardless of whether you're experiencing noticeable respiratory symptoms, instead of deciding on your own whether to take a particular medication.

In some cases, your physician may need to step up your medication to obtain better control of your symptoms, while in other instances, your doctor may recommend stepping down your level of medication if you've been able to consistently achieve good control of your symptoms. (See Chapter 2 for details on the stepwise approach to asthma management.)

Tracking your asthma condition

Because the frequency and character of your symptoms are liable to change throughout your lifetime, your doctor needs to assess your condition on a regular basis, through lung-function tests (usually with spirometry), as well as by evaluating your peak expiratory flow rate, or PEFR (see Chapter 2). This enables your physician to determine whether your current treatment plan is optimal for your current condition, or if it requires adjustment.

Your asthma condition and severity level may also require adjustment due to factors such as:

✔ Seasonal changes, especially those that involve sudden variations in climate and weather, as well as increases or decreases in pollen and mold counts.

✔ Moving to a new building, neighborhood, city, and/or region, which can result in exposure to different types and levels of allergens and irritants.

> ✔ Occupational changes, which may expose you to different types and levels of allergens and irritants.

> ✔ Change in exercise and activity patterns.

> ✔ Change in medical condition, especially if it requires the use of a medication not previously used that has the potential to cause an adverse drug interaction. Consult with your physician about any other prescription or over-the-counter (OTC) medications you may be already taking or may think of taking for other medical conditions, even for relief of minor aches and pains. In some cases, adverse drug interactions can occur between these products and your prescribed asthma medications.

Regular medical visits also enable your doctor to evaluate your inhaler/nebulizer technique (see "Inhalers and Nebulizers," later in this chapter). Your doctor will want to make sure that you derive the maximum benefit from the medication administered by your delivery device.

Effective pharmacotherapy can help you achieve the following goals in managing your asthma:

> ✔ Preventing and controlling your symptoms

> ✔ Reducing the frequency and severity of episodes

> ✔ Reversing your airway obstruction and maintaining improved lung function

Knowing Different Medications

Asthma pharmacotherapy involves two basic classes of medications. These medications are

> ✔ **Long-term control medications:** Doctors prescribe these products as part of a regular, preventive regimen (most often with daily doses) to achieve and control the underlying

airway inflammation that characterizes asthma. For this reason, many of the products in this class are sometimes referred to as *anti-inflammatory drugs* or *controlling drugs*.

✔ **Quick-relief medications:** At times, you may need these products — often called *rescue drugs* or *relieving drugs* — to provide prompt relief of severe and sudden airway constriction and airflow obstruction that can occur when your symptoms unexpectedly worsen.

Your doctor may prescribe products from both classes as part of your long-term asthma management program. The specific combination that your doctor prescribes depends on your asthma's severity and other factors, such as:

✔ **Your age.** Doses and products for infants, toddlers, children under 12, and the elderly often vary from those doses and products that doctors prescribe for children over 12 and adults.

✔ **Your medical history and physical condition.** For example, your doctor may adjust dosages and/or products if you're pregnant or nursing.

✔ **Any other ailments that may affect you, as well as other medications you may take to treat those conditions.** Letting your doctor know about any and all medications you may be using (including OTC ones for minor aches and pains, as well as vitamin supplements and herbal remedies) is essential in order to avoid potential adverse interactions between those products and the asthma medications your doctor may prescribe.

✔ **Any sensitivities you may have to particular drugs or to certain ingredients in the formulations of particular medications.** Some patients may experience tremors or jitteriness when using an older bronchodilator, such as albuterol (Proventil, Ventolin). However, these patients may experience fewer adverse side effects from a newer, improved broncholdilating formulation, such as levalbuterol (Xopenex) and will therefore be more likely to adhere to their asthma medication regimen.

Long-term medications

If used in an appropriate, consistent manner, long-term control medications can reduce existing airway inflammation and may also help prevent further inflammation. However, your doctor should make sure you understand that these types of drugs aren't advisable for rescue relief of a severe asthma episode. For this reason, your asthma management plan should also include a prescribed quick-relief medication (most often a quick-relief bronchodilator, as I explain in "Quick-relief products," later in this chapter).

Long-term control medications include the following:

✔ Anti-inflammatory drugs, such as inhaled corticosteroids (beclomethasone, budesonide, ciclesonide, flunisolide, fluticasone, mometasone, triamcinolone), oral corticosteroids (methylprednisolone, prednisolone, prednisone), and inhaled mast cell stabilizers (cromolyn, nedocromil). These drugs are available in metered-dose inhaler (MDI), dry-powder inhaler (DPI), or compressor-driven nebulizer (CDN) formulations.

✔ Long-acting bronchodilators, such as inhaled salmeterol, formoterol, and oral forms of albuterol. Although most long-acting bronchodilators require at least 10 to 30 minutes to begin providing relief and four to six hours to reach full effect, a newer DPI formulation of formoterol (Foradil), approved by the FDA in 2001, starts working in most patients within one to three minutes.

✔ A combination of the inhaled corticosteroid fluticasone with the long-acting bronchodilator salmeterol, approved by the FDA in 2000. This product, available under the brand name Advair Diskus, treats both airway constriction and inflammation and is one of the most commonly prescribed asthma medications in the U.S.

✔ Sustained release methylxanthine bronchodilators, such as oral theophylline.

✔ Leukotriene modifiers, such as oral montelukast, zafirlukast, and zileuton, available as tablets. If your doctor decides that this category of drugs is suitable for your condition, you may benefit from the ease and convenience of taking tablets, which may help you more effectively adhere to the pharmacotherapy aspect of your asthma management plan. (The FDA has also approved montelukast in pediatric formulations as chewable tablets and oral granules for young children and babies.)

✔ Anti-IgE antibodies, which represent an exciting new development in asthma treatment. Omalizumab/rhuMAb-E25 (Xolair), which physicians administer by injection, is the first drug in this class to be approved by the FDA.

Quick-relief products

Quick-relief drugs, also known as *rescue medications,* promptly reverse acute airflow obstruction and relieve constricted airways during an asthma episode. Your doctor may also prescribe a quick-relief product, such as an inhaled beta$_2$-adrenergic bronchodilator, prior to exercise to prevent symptoms of exercise-induced asthma, or EIA. Quick-relief medications include

✔ **Short-acting beta$_2$-adrenergic bronchodilators.** These adrenaline-like drugs work by rapidly relaxing the smooth muscles in your airways, causing your airways to open, usually within five minutes of inhaling the medication. Inhaled or aerosol forms of these drugs provide the most effective, prompt relief of acute bronchospasms, and many doctors consider beta$_2$-adrenergic bronchodilators the medication of choice for treating asthma symptoms that suddenly worsen and for preventing EIA. Drugs in this class include albuterol (Proventil, Ventolin), bitolterol (Tornalate), metaproterenol (Alupent), pirbuterol (Maxair), and terbutaline (Brethaire, Brethine, Bricanyl). A recently approved new version (single isomer) of albuterol known as *levalbuterol* (Xopenex), a short-acting beta$_2$-adrenergic bronchodilator, is available in nebulizer (CDN) formulations for patients 6 and older.

✔ **Anticholinergics, which may provide added relief when combined with inhaled short-acting beta$_2$-adrenergic bronchodilators.** These drugs block *acetylcholine* (a neurotransmitter that stimulates mucus production) and therefore help reduce mucus in your airways. These drugs also relax the smooth muscle around the lungs' large and medium airways. Ipratropium bromide (Atrovent) is the most widely used anticholinergic in the U.S. and is usually prescribed in combination with short-acting beta$_2$-adrenergic bronchodilators to dilate your airways.

✔ **Oral corticosteroids, also referred to as systemic corticosteroids.** Doctors prescribe these for use in asthma attacks in addition to their use as long-acting medications. During moderate-to-severe asthma episodes, your doctor may use oral corticosteroids to rapidly gain control over worsening symptoms. In such cases, oral corticosteroids can help your other quick-relief medications work more effectively, resulting in a more rapid reversal or reduction of airway inflammation, speeding recovery, and reducing the rate of relapse. Because prolonged use of oral corticosteroids can lead to adverse systemic side effects, doctors typically prescribe these drugs only as a last resort, and discontinue them (by gradual tapering) as soon as symptoms are under control.

Taking medications before surgery

Anesthesia administered during surgery may depress lung functions, so make sure your surgeon is aware of your asthma and the medications you take to control it. (Your surgeon should evaluate both your lung functions and medication use prior to surgery.)

Your doctor may prescribe a short course of oral corticosteroids to improve your lung function starting just prior to surgery. If you've taken oral corticosteroids within the six months prior to surgery, your doctor may also prescribe intravenous hydrocortisone on a set schedule during surgery, with a rapid taper of the dose within 24 hours after your procedure.

Inhalers and Nebulizers

If your medication doesn't go where it's supposed to go, you don't benefit from it. One unique aspect of treating a respiratory condition is that the proper use of an inhaler is as important as the medication itself in the inhaler: The objective is to get the medication to the area of your lungs where it can work most effectively.

Advantages of delivering drugs into your lungs with inhaled delivery systems include the following:

- ✔ You can more effectively administer higher concentrations of medication into your airways.

- ✔ You can reduce the risk of systemic side effects that may occur when you use oral forms of these medications.

- ✔ You receive relief from inhaled drugs faster than with oral products.

Using a metered-dose inhaler

An MDI consists of a canister of pressurized medication that fits into a plastic actuator sleeve and connects to a mouthpiece. An MDI propels medication at more than 60 miles per hour, and that medication needs to make a sharp turn to effectively get into the airways of your lungs. Therefore, most of the medication sprayed from the MDI never even reaches your lungs. For example, the spray can coat your mouth, the end of your tongue, or the back of your throat. In the best-case scenario, your small airways receive only 10 to 20 percent of the inhaled drug.

Millions of asthmatics breathe easier thanks to inhalers, but properly using these devices is crucial to their success. Many people experience difficulty controlling their asthma because they use inhalers incorrectly.

When prescribing your inhaled medication, your physician should instruct you on how to properly use an MDI. She also should review your inhaler technique at subsequent office visits. Here are some important instructions that apply to using most MDI products:

1. **Remove the cap and hold the encased inhaler upright.**

2. **Shake the inhaler.**

3. **Tilt your head back slightly and breathe out slowly.**

4. **Depending on your physician's specific instructions, open your mouth with your head 1 to 2 inches away from the inhaler or position the inhaler in your mouth.**

5. **Press down on the inhaler to release medication as you start inhaling or within the first second of inhaling; continue inhaling as you press down on your inhaler.** Breathe in slowly through your mouth, not your nose, for three to five seconds. Press your inhaler only once while you're inhaling

(one breath for each puff). Make sure to breathe evenly and deeply.

6. **Hold your breath for ten seconds to allow the medicine to reach deep into your lungs.**

7. **Repeat puffs as your prescription dictates.** Waiting one minute between puffs may permit the second puff to reach into the airways of your lungs better.

Two important factors that can affect the dosage you receive from your MDI include the following:

✔ **Loss of prime:** Keeping too many backup inhalers around can lead to infrequent inhaler activation and *loss of prime,* which occurs when the inhaler's propellant evaporates or escapes from the metering chamber after days or weeks of nonuse. If you haven't used an inhaler recently, waste a puff of medication (often less than a full dose) into the air before inhaling your first dose to ensure that you receive the full potency of your medication.

✔ **Tail-off:** In a misguided attempt to economize, many inhaler users try to squeeze every last drop of medication from their MDIs. However, research indicates that this practice may actually contribute to the documented rise in asthma deaths and poor quality of life for some people with asthma because of a phenomenon known as *tail-off.* As an MDI reaches its empty stage, dose reliability becomes increasingly unpredictable. Therefore, don't use your MDI beyond the labeled number of doses, even if you think that some medication remains.

Many patients have found that the recently developed Maxair Autohaler, formulated to deliver pirbuterol (a short-acting beta$_2$-adrenergic bronchodilator), is a simpler, user-friendly way of delivering medication to the airways compared to many other MDIs. That's mainly because the Autohaler is the only breath-activated MDI approved by the FDA, and requires less coordination to use. The Autohaler also doesn't require the use of a holding chamber, or spacer (see the next section).

Given the more sophisticated design and effectiveness of the Autohaler and of various dry-powder inhalers as well as the recently approved Advair Diskus (which I discuss later in this section), you may wonder why generic MDIs continue to be prescribed.

The reason for that is simple: dollars and cents. A bottom-line attitude has taken over the health-care industry, and too often, in the name of cost containment, physicians prescribe low-cost generics rather than brand-name products. Many asthma patients may not be receiving the treatment they really require because too often their physicians prescribe generic medications rather than costlier brand-name products, such as the Autohaler, which feature more advanced drug for-mulations and easier-to-use inhalation systems.

Using holding chambers

Doctors recommend *holding chambers* (also known as *spacers*) for younger children and people who can't use an MDI correctly. This hollow device extends the space between the opening of the inhaler and your mouth. It traps and suspends particles of medication as the inhaler releases them, allowing you to inhale your dose over a span of one to six breaths, depending on the par-ticular device you use. Use a holding chamber when taking inhaled corticosteroids with an MDI to minimize the possibility of developing an oral yeast infection and to improve delivery of the medication to your lungs.

Holding chambers come in various shapes and sizes. Several of these devices (such as AeroChamber and E-Z Spacer) have both a mouthpiece for adults, as shown in Figure 5-1, and a mask for infants and small children, as shown in Figure 5-2.

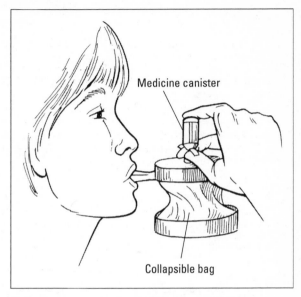

Medicine canister

Collapsible bag

Figure 5-1: An adult using an MDI with a mouthpiece.

Using a dry-powder inhaler

DPIs dispense medication in a dry-powder formulation. DPIs come in different shapes and sizes and can deliver bronchodilators as well as anti-inflammatory medications. In recent years, the FDA has approved DPI formulations of the four following long-acting drugs:

✔ Budesonide, an inhaled corticosteroid, distributed in the United States as Pulmicort Turbuhaler

> ✔ Fluticasone, also an inhaled corticosteroid,
> available as Flovent Rotadisk to be used with
> the Diskhaler device
>
> ✔ Salmeterol, a long-acting bronchodilator, mar-
> keted as Serevent Diskus
>
> ✔ Fluticasone and salmeterol in combination, mar-
> keted as Advair Diskus

DPIs are easy to use and very effective, if you operate
them properly. The medication particles in the dry
powder are so small that they can easily reach the
tiniest airways. Keep in mind that, unlike most MDIs,
with a few types of DPIs, you may not taste or feel the
medication when using the device. If you've administered the medication properly, however, you will
receive its benefit.

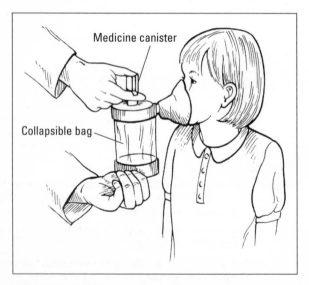

Figure 5-2: A child using an MDI with a mask.

Specific benefits of using a DPI include the following:

✔ Children as young as 4 can use these devices.

✔ For people who have poor MDI technique or who have difficulty coordinating the steps required for properly inhaling medication from an MDI, a DPI is often an excellent alternative, especially for kids.

✔ One inhalation from a DPI often provides the same dosage as two puffs of a comparable medication from an MDI.

✔ Because some DPIs have dose counters, you can easily tell when your inhaler is almost empty.

✔ Cold temperatures don't reduce the effectiveness of DPIs.

✔ DPIs don't use chlorofluorocarbons (CFCs), so they don't damage the planet's ozone layer.

Although DPIs don't require using a holding chamber, you still need to use your DPI in a specific way. Because every DPI works a little differently, make sure you know how to use the one your doctor prescribes. As with an MDI, your doctor should instruct you on how to properly use your DPI and should review your inhaler technique at subsequent office visits. The following are important, general instructions on the proper use of most DPIs:

1. **Follow the manufacturer's instructions to prime your DPI and then load a prescribed dose of the dry-powder medication.**

2. **Breathe out slowly and completely (usually for three to five seconds).**

3. **Put your mouth on the mouthpiece and inhale deeply and forcefully.**

4. **Hold your breath for ten seconds and then exhale slowly.**

5. **Repeat the procedure as outlined by your physician until you've taken the correct number of doses.**

In addition to the previous steps, keep these points in mind to obtain the most benefit from your DPI:

✔ **Your DPI is breath-activated.** That means you can control the rate at which you inhale the dry powder. However, you do need to inhale with sufficient force (minimal flow rate) to assure delivery of the medication to the smallest airways of your lungs. To be truly effective, using a DPI requires closing your mouth tightly around the inhaler's mouthpiece and inhaling steadily, deeply, and forcefully.

✔ **Make sure the dry powder in your DPI stays dry to avoid caking or clumping, which can affect the dose's reliability.** For DPIs with caps, always replace the cap after using the product. Don't ever wash a DPI that still contains medication.

✔ **In contrast with the operation of an MDI, you don't need to shake your DPI just before using it in order to assure delivery of the proper dose.** Shaking some DPIs can result in losing dry powder.

Using a multidose-powder inhaler

Advair, a recently approved combination of fluticasone (an inhaled corticosteroid) with salmeterol (a long-acting beta$_2$-adrenergic bronchodilator), is formulated in a new type of delivery device known as a Diskus. As with other DPIs, the Diskus is breath-activated, and for the majority of patients, it's easier to use than most MDIs.

The FDA approved this product, the first of its kind, to treat both the underlying inflammation that characterizes asthma and the airway constriction that often results from episodes of respiratory symptoms. Evidence suggests that using Advair Diskus usually reduces airway inflammation within one or two weeks (sometimes longer in certain cases), while the medication's bronchodilation effects are usually felt within 30 to 60 minutes. However, remember that Advair Diskus isn't a replacement for a quick-relief drug that your doctor prescribes for you to use if your respiratory symptoms worsen.

Important advantages of Advair Diskus include these:

✔ Each dose of Advair is effective for up to 12 hours. The normal dosage is one inhalation twice per day (for patients 12 years and older): once in the morning and once at night. This medication schedule is often more practical for patients than most MDI medications. As a result, patients using Advair Diskus are liable to be more successful in adhering to an asthma management plan.

✔ Using the Diskus requires far less coordination than most MDIs.

✔ The built-in Diskus dose counter lets you keep track of every dose.

If your physician prescribes Advair Diskus for you, make sure she explains the proper use of it. The following are important, general instructions when using the Diskus:

1. **While holding the device in one hand, place the thumb of your other hand on the device's thumb grip and push away until the mouthpiece appears and snaps into position.**

2. **Hold the Diskus in a level, horizontal position with the mouthpiece facing you and slide the lever away from you as far as it goes until it clicks.** The "click" means the Diskus is ready for use.

3. **Exhale, while holding the Diskus level but away from your mouth (never exhale into the Diskus mouthpiece).**

4. **Place the mouthpiece to your lips, and breathe in quickly and deeply through the Diskus (don't breathe in through your nose).**

5. **Remove the Diskus from your mouth and hold your breath for about ten seconds or as long as you find comfortable; exhale slowly through your mouth.**

6. **Close the Diskus when you have completed taking a dose.** To do so, place your thumb once again on the thumb grip and slide it back toward you as far as it goes. The Diskus clicks shut, and the lever returns to its original position. The device is ready for your next dose, which you should take in about 12 hours (unless your doctor has advised you differently).

7. **After taking your Diskus dose, rinse your mouth with water without swallowing.**

Beyond the previous general Advair Diskus instructions, keep the following points in mind to get the most out of this medication:

✔ Don't advance the lever more than once when preparing your dose, and don't play with the lever.

✔ Avoid tilting the Diskus when using it. Only use it in a level, horizontal position.

✔ Never try to take the Diskus apart.

✔ Always keep the Diskus dry. Never wash any part of the device, including the mouthpiece.

Using nebulizers

A *nebulizer* is an air compressor connected to a generator. Nebulizers deliver medication as a mist that is easy to inhale, which often brings rapid symptom relief. These medication-delivery systems, sometimes known as *breathing machines,* are especially useful when a child is too young or too sick to use other devices. In addition to standard, home plug-in models, you can purchase portable nebulizers with battery packs or cigarette lighter adapters to use in a vehicle.

Although at times a bit more expensive in terms of the initial purchase price, the newer jet nebulizers are preferable to older units. The slight cost difference between these newer nebulizers and their precursor evaporates after patients begin using the more modern machines and realize how much more effectively they deliver medication throughout the airways.

Doctors typically recommend jet nebulizers as the delivery device for administering Pulmicort Respules, a commonly prescribed CDN formulation of the inhaled corticosteroid drug budesonide.

Doctors may prescribe nebulizer therapy for adults to reduce or eliminate hospital or emergency room visits, especially for severe persistent asthma sufferers. Many nebulizer users find that the device allows them more effective relief than metered-dose inhalers. Therefore, if you're experiencing sudden-onset, severe asthma attacks on a frequent basis, you may benefit greatly from having a nebulizer prescribed for home use.

Remember these general guidelines when using a nebulizer with a mouthpiece:

✔ Place your mouth over the mouthpiece and breathe in and out.

✔ Breathe through your mouth and not your nose. You or your child can use a facemask that covers the mouth and nose with the nebulizer. Some nebulizer manufacturers also offer colorful, kid-friendly pediatric masks. These masks usually feature animal shapes and can help in making the process of using a nebulizer more attractive — even fun in some cases — for young children.

✔ Have an extra nebulizer mask on hand when using the device, especially if you're administering the medication to a young child. (If you have a young child, you can probably imagine any number of reasons why that extra mask might come in handy.)

✔ When using a nebulizer on your child, don't "blow by" or mist the medication in your child's face. A nebulizer requires a closed system to provide effective treatment.

✔ Use all the medication in your nebulizer. (Doing so normally takes 7 to 15 minutes, depending on the type of nebulizer you're using.)

Cleaning your system

Rinse your MDI, holding chamber, and nebulizer daily and wash them weekly with a mild detergent to keep them clean and free of medication build-up. Don't use harsh chemicals in washing them, and make sure to follow the manufacturer's instructions for maintenance and care. Also, don't forget any MDIs that have been sitting in a drawer, backpack, briefcase, or handbag for a long time.

Remember to always keep the cap on your inhaler when you're not using it. If the cap accidentally becomes dislodged, make sure that you properly clean your inhaler before using it again.

Chapter 6

Ten Tips for Traveling with Asthma

*I*f only airlines could lose your asthma the way they sometimes lose your baggage. Imagine if you could leave your wheezing instead of your heart in San Francisco. And wouldn't waking up in the city that never sleeps because the Big Apple stirs you to the very core — instead of an asthma episode interrupting a good night's rest — be nice?

Of course, getting away from asthma isn't that easy. Think of asthma, and often-related conditions, such as *allergic rhinitis* (hay fever), as constant companions. Wherever you may roam, these conditions are along for the ride. Knowing how to control symptoms is vital to ensuring that no matter what else may go wrong during your travel, your respiratory condition won't complicate or ruin your plans.

Planning a Safe, Healthy Trip

A key element in proper travel planning is avoiding places where you know pollens, dander, tobacco smoke, or other allergens and irritants may be prevalent and could, depending on your specific sensitivities, trigger your respiratory and/or allergy symptoms. The following points are guidelines for preventing problems frequently associated with these triggers:

✔ **Dander:** Beware of visiting or staying in homes with cats, dogs, and other animals, including rabbits, birds, and gerbils and other domesticated rodents. Even if the animal lover removes the pet from the area, you can still suffer an adverse reaction because of the residual dander and/or hair in the room. Horseback riding also may not be advisable. Consult your doctor about preventive medications (and see Chapters 3 and 4).

✔ **Food allergens:** The foods that trigger allergic reactions most frequently in adults with food hypersensitivities include fish, shellfish, peanuts, and tree nuts. For children, the most common triggers are milk, eggs, peanuts, tree nuts, fish, soy, and wheat. Because of the swiftness and severity with which a food allergy reaction can strike (especially with peanuts), be especially vigilant in avoiding these triggers when traveling. In particular, if you or your child is sensitive to peanuts and you're planning to travel where these seemingly harmless legumes are a regular part of local cuisine (many parts of East Asia, for example), ask your doctor about additional precautions you can take. Although you can clearly identify peanuts in many dishes, they may be a hidden part of the cooking process itself in many cases (for example, foods cooked alongside dishes prepared with peanut products). When in doubt, avoid local fare in these parts of the world, rather than risk reactions such as an asthma attack, hives, or worse yet, a potentially life-threatening case of anaphylaxis.

✔ **Ragweed:** Avoiding travel to the eastern half of the United States and Canada from mid-August through October is probably advisable (assuming you don't already live there) if you're sensitized to ragweed pollen. If you must travel to those areas during ragweed season (see Chapter 4), ask your physician about preventive medications that you can take to keep your symptoms under control. Also, the National Allergy Bureau (NAB) of the American Academy of Allergy, Asthma, and Immunology (AAAAI) has seasonal allergen maps that chart the prevalence of allergenic pollens, as well as several other allergens around the country throughout the year. Check out the NAB Web site at www.aaaai.org/nab or call 414-272-6071. (See Chapter 4 for more information on pollens.)

Adjusting Treatment for Travel

Prevention is the key to a safe and trouble-free trip, which usually means consulting your physician ahead of time to evaluate your asthma management and to make any advisable adjustments, based on where and when you're going and what you'll be doing while traveling. You may need to adjust your medication because of increased exposures to triggers. In addition, remember that changes in time zones may affect the dosage schedule of some medications you're taking (for any ailment, not just asthma).

You'll also need to make sure that you'll be able to stick with the program that your physician advises. If possible, get a letter from your doctor summarizing your medical history, as well as the treatments and medications you're currently taking. If you're at risk of acute asthma or allergy attacks, ask your physician about wearing a MedicAlert pendant on your wrist or around your neck.

Taking Medications and Other Essentials

Make sure you have all your necessary medical supplies, devices, and prescriptions with you when traveling. Keep these items in your carry-on bag. After you arrive at your destination, keep your essentials with you instead of leaving them in your hotel room (or other accommodation) when you're out and about. If you need to leave your medications in the room, make sure you store them in a safe, secure location, such as the room safe or in a locked suitcase, instead of leaving them out on the bathroom countertop.

Keep medications in their original containers and never mix pills of different types into one receptacle. By keeping them in their original containers, you'll have the proper dosage information readily available, which is especially important if someone else needs to administer your medication to you. Also, if you're traveling internationally, customs officials are generally less suspicious of pills and capsules in their original containers.

If you or your child uses a nebulizer at home, ask your doctor about taking one with you on your trip. If you're traveling overseas, don't

forget to bring whatever adapters and convert-
ers (available in most luggage, electronics,
and travel stores) you may need in order to use
your domestic devices in different countries.
The electric current in many other parts of the
world is 220 volts rather than the 110 volts that
is standard in the United States and Canada. If
you have a portable nebulizer, don't forget extra
batteries.

Getting Medications and Medical Help Abroad

 Ask your doctor about special medical considerations for specific countries and areas. Some
countries require that you take certain vaccine
shots before your visit. As for medications, don't
assume that every place you visit has pharma-
cies stocked with the supplies you need. Write
down both the brand names of your medications
and their generic names. In a pinch, having both
names available may allow a local pharmacist to
find what you need.

When planning your trip, you may want to obtain a
booklet that lists qualified, English-speaking physicians in just about every country of the world. The
International Association for Medical Assistance to
Travelers (IAMAT), a voluntary organization based in
Canada, offers this booklet. You can contact them in
the United States at 716-754-4883 or via their Web site
at www.iamat.org for further information.

Also, if you're a U.S. citizen, the U.S. State Department's
American Citizens Services can provide help in case
of an emergency. Call the State Department's Hotline

for American Travelers, 202-647-5225, or check the State Department's Web site, www.state.gov, before your departure to receive information on contacting U.S. embassies and consulates for assistance with medical matters.

Flying with Allergens and Irritants

Sad to say, but your fellow airplane passengers may make you sick. Studies show that airplane passenger cabins are some of the worst indoor dust mite and animal dander sites. Because airliners are tightly sealed environments that often lack adequate air filtering or cleaning, they often concentrate sky-high quantities of allergens and irritants that hundreds, even thousands, of passengers constantly track in with them. So be advised: Your seat may already be occupied by frequent-flier allergens.

Many airplane seats house thriving colonies of dust mites and their allergenic waste products. In addition, although all U.S., Canadian, and many European flights ban smoking anywhere on the aircraft (and in most parts of airport terminals), some international flights still allow smoking.

 If exposure to tobacco smoke triggers your asthma symptoms, find out as much as possible about an air carrier's smoking policies. If your travel includes flying an airline that permits smoking, try to get seating as far away from the smoking section as possible.

Take my advice when you're planning air travel:

✔ **Pack your medications in a carry-on bag so they're immediately available in the event of a serious asthma episode and/or allergic reaction and in case the airline loses your luggage.** (You want to avoid finding yourself in strange territory without your medications.)

✔ **Stay hydrated during your flight.** Avoid alcohol and drink plenty of water. Not only does drinking water help minimize potential asthma and allergy problems, but it also can put a dent in whatever jet lag you may otherwise develop.

✔ **If you have the opportunity/financial ability, consider upgrading to first or business class.** If available, the leather seats may be less likely to harbor allergy triggers, and at the very least, you'll give yourself more breathing (and leg) room.

Considering Allergy Shots

When you're traveling, I usually recommend transferring your immunotherapy (allergy shots) program to another location only if you'll be gone at least a month or more (if you're a snowbird from the North wintering in southern California or southern Florida, for example). If you'll be gone for a month or more, ask your physician for a referral to a doctor in the area where you'll be staying and have that physician administer your shots in a medical facility.

Although practices vary in different areas of the U.S. and the world, don't give yourself allergy shots. The risk, although low, of a bad reaction or even anaphylactic shock means you need qualified medical personnel around you, just in case.

When visiting the physician in the new location, bring your allergy serum (vaccine) vials in a refrigerated or ice-insulated pack, and make sure you have clear written instructions from your doctor regarding your dose.

Reducing Trigger Exposures in Hotels and Motels

Tobacco smoke and its lingering traces can cause problems, especially outside the United States or Canada, where hotels and other accommodations are less likely to restrict smoking. Wherever you stay, reserve a room on a smoke-free floor. Likewise, if feathers pose a potential allergy problem for you, bring your own pillow and pillowcase (see Chapter 4).

Inspect the room before you occupy it, looking for signs of animal hair, dirty air vents, dust, or mold. If you find evidence suggesting that staying in the room will lead to breathing problems, ask for another room that appears safer and more comfortable. In some cases, your doctor may advise bringing along a portable HEPA air filter system (see Chapter 3). Check to see whether your hotel offers allergy-free rooms, which may even come with HEPA filters and allergy covers on the mattresses.

Avoiding Food Allergies

In your travels, you may come into contact with foods to which you have an allergy (not just an intolerance). In some cases, the menu reveals all you need to know about potentially problematic ingredients. But more often than not, you need to ask a lot of questions about the cuisine and how it's prepared. Don't be rude, but definitely don't be shy.

You may need to do more than simply determine that a particular dish doesn't contain foods to which you're allergic. For example, in many restaurants, various dishes are all prepared on the same grill. In this case, if you're allergic to shellfish, for example, make sure that the cooking surface and utensils used to prepare your food haven't also been previously used to prepare shellfish. If they have, allergens from the shellfish may end up in your meal, potentially causing a distressful dining experience.

If your food hypersensitivities put you at risk for anaphylaxis, wear a MedicAlert pendant or bracelet. Also ask your doctor about prescribing an epinephrine kit such as an EpiPen, and be sure to carry it with you.

Finding Help in Case of Emergencies

Although the local hospital probably isn't at the top of your sightseeing list, find out the location of the nearest medical facility equipped to treat you in case of a serious adverse allergic reaction or severe asthma episode. Knowing where the closest help is available can help ensure that you get effective treatment if you experience a life-threatening reaction.

Depending on your destination, you can easily obtain local hospital locations from the organizations that I list earlier in this chapter (see "Getting Medications and Medical Help Abroad"), your doctor, or your travel agent. In some cases, you may need to do more homework; your health and safety are worth the effort.

Traveling with Your Asthmatic Child

 When traveling with a child who has asthma, many of the same considerations that adults must contend with also apply:

- ✔ **Pack two containers of all medications, and make sure that you've labeled them properly.** Keep one container as a carry-on with you, and keep the other in a purse, backpack, or briefcase.

- ✔ **Obtain a MedicAlert bracelet or necklace for your child to wear.** If you're not around, emergency medical personnel will immediately know what to do about your child's condition.

- ✔ **Show your child how to pack his or her medications properly.** In addition to preparing your child for trips that he or she may take without you, this lesson can also help your youngster find out more about managing his or her condition appropriately.

- ✔ **Take at least two epinephrine kits (such as an EpiPen or EpiPen Jr. for children under 66 pounds) if your child is at risk for anaphylaxis to ensure that you'll always have one at hand.** Make sure that you and/or your child (depending on the youngster's age) know how to use the kit. You should receive instructions on the proper use of the injector in your doctor's office, rather than waiting for a potential emergency to figure it out.

- ✔ **Ask questions about meals.** If your child has peanut allergies, be especially vigilant on airplanes (particularly with the contents of those appealingly packaged snack bags), where peanuts can be as common as delayed flights.

Diet, Health & Fitness Titles from For Dummies

For Dummies books help keep you healthy and fit. Whatever your health & fitness needs, turn to Dummies books first.

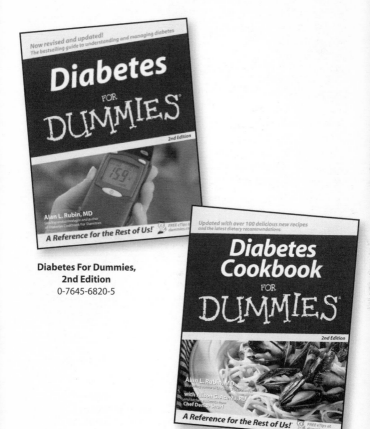

**Diabetes For Dummies,
2nd Edition**
0-7645-6820-5

**Diabetes Cookbook For Dummies,
2nd Edition**
0-7645-8450-2

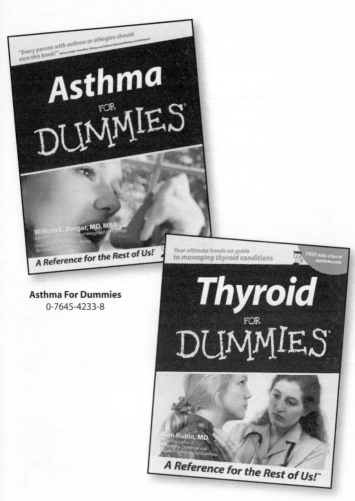

Asthma For Dummies
0-7645-4233-8

Thyroid For Dummies
0-7645-5385-2

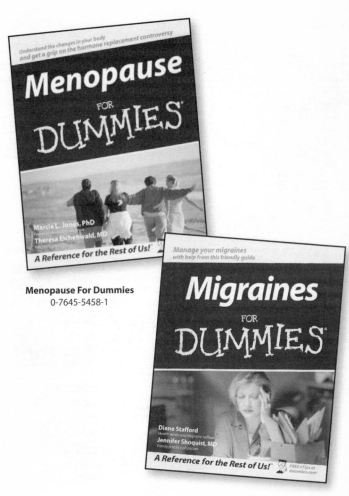

Menopause For Dummies
0-7645-5458-1

Migraines For Dummies
0-7645-5485-9

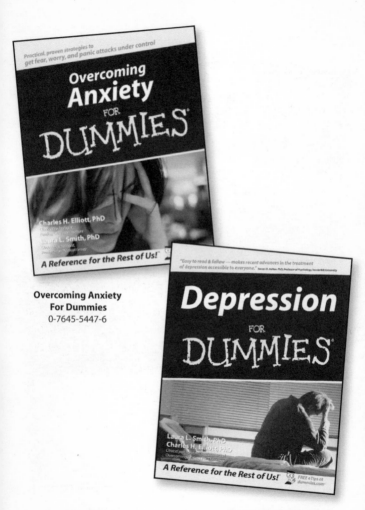

**Overcoming Anxiety
For Dummies**
0-7645-5447-6

Depression For Dummies
0-7645-3900-0

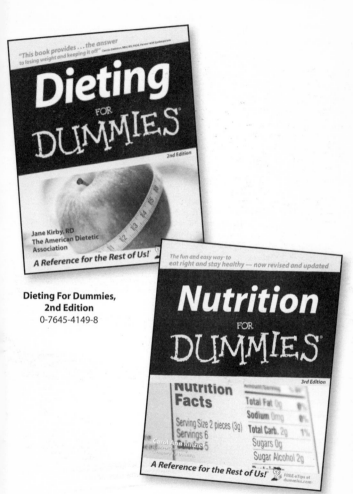

**Dieting For Dummies,
2nd Edition**
0-7645-4149-8

**Nutrition For Dummies,
3rd Edition**
0-7645-4082-3

After you've read the Pocket Edition, look for the original Dummies book on the topic. The handy Contents at a Glance below highlights the information you'll get when you purchase a copy of *Asthma For Dummies* – available wherever books are sold, or visit dummies.com.

Contents at a Glance